Health
Ministries

Health Ministries

A Primer for Clergy and Congregations

DEBORAH L. PATTERSON

THE
PILGRIM
PRESS
Cleveland

*To my colleagues at the Deaconess Foundation,
Deaconess Parish Nurse Ministries,
and the International Parish Nurse Resource Center,
health ministers all,
and to my dear family,
with heartfelt thanks.*

In memory of Norella V. Huggins.

The Pilgrim Press
700 Prospect Avenue
Cleveland, Ohio 44115-1100
thepilgrimpress.com

© 2008 by Deborah Patterson

All rights reserved. Published 2008

❀ Printed in the United States of America on acid-free paper that contains post-consumer fiber.

12 11 10 09 08   5 4 3 2

Library of Congress Cataloging-in-Publication Data
Patterson, Deborah L., 1956–
    Health ministries : a primer for clergy and congregations / Deborah L. Patterson.
        p. ; cm.
    ISBN 978-0-8298-1791-1 (alk. paper)
    1. Parish nursing. 2. Pastoral medicine – Catholic Church. 3. Church work with the sick – Catholic Church. I. Title.
    [DNLM: 1. Nursing. 2. Religion. 3. Community Health Nursing. 4. Pastoral Care. WY 145 P317h 2007]
    RT120.P37P386 2007
    610.73′43 – dc22
                                                                        2007045235

Healing is impossible in loneliness;
it is the opposite of loneliness.
Conviviality is healing.
To be healed we must come
with all the other creatures
to the feast of Creation.
                    —Wendell Berry

Contents

Preface and Acknowledgments

The *Washington Post* recently reported that Baby Boomers appear to be less healthy than their parents were at the same age. Researchers from the University of Texas at Austin found that "the trend seems to be that people are not as healthy as they approach retirement as they were in older generations." The study reports that "boomers tend to report more stress than earlier generations — from their jobs, their commutes, taking care of their parents and their kids — all of which can take a physical toll, which is compounded by having less support from extended families and communities."

Lisa Berkman of the Harvard School of Public Health says, "People are working two jobs. They are not sleeping as much. They're experiencing more job insecurity. They have less time to take care of themselves. They are more socially isolated."[1] Didn't we recently see the results of isolation in the despair of a young student at Virginia Tech?

Thirty years ago, German theologian Dorothee Sölle published a book about the "inner journey." Translated later under the title *Death by Bread Alone,* the book considered religious experiences, texts, and their interpretations. Sölle discussed our need for liberation. Like Jesus, who, when tempted, replied, "Man does not live by bread alone," she reminds us that true life lies in finding meaning and purpose, having compassion for those who are suffering, and creating a sense of community with others.

Farmer, poet, and novelist Wendell Berry writes, "I believe that the community — in the fullest sense: a place and all its creatures — is the smallest unit of health and that to speak of the health of an isolated individual is a contradiction in terms."[2]

Parish nurses, pastors, and other health ministers have a tremendous opportunity to make a difference in today's world. They see the strain of people taking care of aging parents and children with special needs. They hear the stress of people who work full time but do not have health insurance for themselves and earn too much for their children to be eligible. They know the anxiety of people who struggle with chronic illness. They reach out to people who are longing for meaning, for connection, for hope.

Recently, I heard a statistic that 80 percent of twenty-year-olds in the United States have never been to church (other than to a wedding or funeral). I'm assuming they are not adherents of other faiths, either. What spiritual sustenance are we offering them?

Integrating spirituality and health has been the mission of faith communities for millennia. Finding new ways to make that possible to all generations within changing societies is always a challenge. Yet signs of a new awakening to the church's role in health and wholeness are everywhere — from parish nurses to health clinics to congregations working fervently for health care finance reform. Across the land and around the globe, faith communities are forming a vision of community and healing that can offer sustenance and hope to all.

In this small volume, I hope to convince fellow clergy that parish nursing is a viable ministry with which to support and multiply the many health ministries that already exist within congregations. I also hope to encourage them to grow their current health ministries and explore other options. Most congregations have outreach to hospitals, to nursing homes, and to those who are homebound. Many offer counseling. Some have food pantries, while others provide housing for the homeless.

I would encourage you to read the brief chapters that follow to see how parish nursing might link with your already existing ministries. There are many different models for providing health ministry with the assistance of parish nurses, and one of them may be right for your congregation. If you do not have a nurse who is able to serve in this capacity, many of the ideas in this book can be adapted for use by other health professionals, counselors, teachers, or other church members, in cooperation with local community health resources.

In chapter 2, "Parish Nursing: A Beneficial Partnership for Clergy," I hope to convince you that you have everything to gain, and nothing to lose, by investing some time and resources in exploring this growing ecumenical and interfaith movement.

I would like to take a moment to thank the many parish nurses whom I have had the pleasure of meeting, interviewing, or working with over the past dozen years. In my capacity as executive director of the International Parish Nurse Ministry, I am able to work full time with members of this remarkable profession, as well as with clergy from a wide variety of faith traditions. I am always pleasantly surprised to hear of the many creative ways that pastors and parish nurses have found to serve the members of their congregations, as well as their neighbors, through programming that includes parish nursing. I have included a health ministry story with each chapter, and I would like to thank the many people who shared their perspectives, some of which appeared earlier in the pages of *Parish Nurse Perspectives,* a quarterly print publication of the International Parish Nurse Resource Center. I am also grateful to the parish nurses and congregations who allowed their ministries to be mentioned and included in this book.

Thank you to Rebecca Grothe, editor of the *Clergy Journal,* in which several of these chapters first appeared in varied forms. Without Rebecca's receptiveness to these topics, this book would not exist today. Thank you also to Kathy Schoonover-Shoffner, PhD, RN, editor of the *Journal of Christian Nursing,* for her commitment to offering a strong voice for the specialty practice of parish nursing, and for first publishing "Eight Advocacy Roles for Parish Nurses," in the January–March 2007 issue. The article appears here as chapter 12 under the title "As You Have done to the Least of These, You Have Done to Me: Health Advocacy." This article is copyrighted by Lippincott, Williams &

Wilkins, whom I would like to thank for permission to reprint it here. Thank you to Patricia Gleich, associate for National Health Ministries at the Presbyterian Church USA, a passionate spirit for health ministry, to my colleagues at the Health Ministries Association, and to the members of the Health Care Task Force of the National Council of the Churches of Christ in the USA. A special thanks to Rev. Eileen W. Lindner, PhD, deputy general secretary for Research and Planning at the NCC, whose groundbreaking research on health ministry in the Congregational Health Ministry Survey Report will prove its importance in the coming years.

Thanks also to the entire staff at The Pilgrim Press, particularly Kim Sadler, editorial director for Educational and Congregational Resources, and to John Eagleson, whose careful attention to detail improved the manuscript greatly.

A special word of thanks to the staff of the Deaconess Foundation in St. Louis for their support of the work of parish nursing and other health ministries, particularly the Reverend Jerry W. Paul, president and CEO of the Deaconess Foundation, as well as Dr. Nesa Joseph, vice president, who provides administrative support to our organization. Both Rev. Paul and Dr. Joseph have a long history both with institutional health care and the wider church in the United States and abroad.

Thank you to the entire board of the Deaconess Parish Nurse Ministries, who have given our organization the support to work on projects such as these. Thank you also to the administrative staff of Deaconess Parish Nurse Ministries, with whom I work each day. I name each of them here, because they have provided great inspiration and support: Alvyne Rethemeyer, Maureen Daniels, Barbara Wehling, Gayle Mason, Eileen McGartland, Sharon Salerno, Karen Howe, and especially Susan Miller, who helped me with my computer and printed several versions of this manuscript.

Thanks to each and every one of the Deaconess parish nurses in the metropolitan St. Louis area, whose ministries touch and bless many, many thousands of people in this community and beyond. You are wise and compassionate healers.

And thanks to you, health ministers all. The fields are white unto harvest. We have much to do.

Notes

1. Rob Stein, "Baby Boomers Appear to Be Less Healthy Than Parents," *Washington Post*, April 20, 2007.

2. "Health Is Membership," as quoted in "Other Voices," in the recent "Health" issue of the journal of the Center for Christian Ethics, entitled *Christian Reflection: A Series in Faith and Ethics* (Waco, Tex.: Baylor University Press, 2007), 61.

One

Called to Preach, Teach, *and* Heal
Health Ministries in the Church

Jesus called his followers to "preach, teach, and heal." Walk into most congregations around the world today on a Sunday morning, and you will likely hear preaching. Walk into most congregations around the world today on a Sunday morning, and you will likely find teaching, through Sunday School, Adult Education, and other settings. However, walk into most congregations around the world today and you are unlikely to find an organized effort at healing beyond that of prayer and pastoral visitation. Health ministry is an attempt to reclaim the leadership role of the church in Christ's ministry of healing in the world. After all, many or the hospitals in the world were started by churches. It is time for the Christian churches to reclaim their voice and vision for healing of body, mind, spirit, community, and creation.

The modern congregational health ministry movement has its roots in the story of a Lutheran pastor, Rev. Dr. Granger E. Westberg. As a young pastor at St. John's Lutheran Church in Bloomington, Illinois, in the early 1940s, Rev. Westberg, who was on the board of Augustana Hospital in Chicago, had an opportunity to serve as a vacation replacement chaplain there for one week — a week that he said changed his life.[1] At that time, the majority of chaplains were elderly clergy who had retired from pastoral ministry. Most worked part time, and few were trained in clinical pastoral education. Typically, a chaplain simply moved from patient to patient, distributing devotional materials and offering prayer. During his short stint at Augustana Hospital, Rev. Westberg was surprised to learn that most of the physicians and some of the nurses did not take the spiritual mission of the hospital seriously. He became convinced, as others did elsewhere, that chaplains needed clinical skills in counseling or other health-related fields if they were to be regarded as competent members of the health care team.

In the months that followed, Rev. Westberg began writing about new, more meaningful roles for chaplains. He argued that competent, well-educated chaplains could help revitalize the church's hospital ministry.

Three years later, when Augustana Hospital needed another chaplain, Rev. Westberg asked to be considered for the position. Since he was a young man with a promising future, most of his colleagues thought his decision to leave pastoral ministry unwise, but he persisted. In 1944, after completing work in clinical pastoral education, Rev. Westberg became the first full-time chaplain at Augustana Hospital, a position he held for eight years.

One of Rev. Westberg's first innovations there was the creation of a course on the relationship between religion and health as part of the nursing curriculum. Although religious studies had been common in nursing schools during the late 1800s, by the 1940s few schools of nursing in Christian hospitals still included more than cursory mention of religion in their curricula. All focus was on science. In fact, it wasn't until the 1990s that an entire chapter on spirituality appeared in a "modern" nursing textbook.[2]

In 1952, Rev. Westberg received a joint appointment in Religion and Health at the University of Chicago in the divinity and medical schools as chaplain of the University of Chicago Clinics and associate professor of pastoral care in the Federated Theological Faculty. This made him the first person at a major university to have such a joint appointment.[3] While there, he advocated and demonstrated wholistic approaches to health care that were firmly grounded in traditional religious and medical practices. He advocated the use of the word "wholistic" (rather than "holistic"), to more closely resemble the word "whole" and to avoid confusion with alternative health care practices that were just beginning to spring up at the time. He wrote:

> There is a great ferment on the West Coast around the general subject of "holistic medicine." Recently, some 3,000 people attended a two-day conference there on holistic medicine, but I sense that they are really not talking about the same thing as we are. They show great enthusiasm for what we might consider "far-out" kinds of health care. I salute them for their willingness to test new ways to get at the cause and cure of illness. However, a number of people are confused by the similarity of our names. I have tried very hard to keep our project within the fold of traditional American medicine and religion.[4]

Westberg saw that the mainline Christian and Jewish faith traditions had a long and proud history as leaders in health care, stating:

> One hundred years ago physicians in this country needed facilities for the care of their very sick patients and turned for help to the Catholics, Protestants and Jews. These groups responded by building magnificent hospitals all over the land, which we now take quite for granted. We are greatly in debt to them for their contributions to health care during these 100 years.
>
> Then the physicians said, "We need schools to train young doctors" and the religious people complied; and again the physicians said, "We need more nurses to provide good health care" and the congregations built nursing schools. Then the church people decided they weren't really needed and left the institutions they built to be run by scientists.
>
> Now physicians again need help, this time in the area of preventative medicine. They know that much illness starts in the home or neighborhood or is related to a person's job. They are wondering if somehow the clergy can help them to get to people in the earlier stages of illness. Perhaps

churches, which are to be found in every community, could be a key factor in providing this help.[5]

It was because of Rev. Westberg's belief that churches were an important resource, long connected to the roots, growth, and development of health care, that he envisioned a new model for care, which started with the Wholistic Health Centers. It is to that development that we now turn.

Wholistic Health Centers

As the first dean of the Institute of Religion at the Texas Medical Center in Houston during the mid-1960s, Rev. Westberg further explored the concept of the parish as a healing community. Later, as professor of practical theology at Wittenberg University's Hamma School of Theology in Springfield, Ohio, Westberg founded a church clinic, with volunteer doctors, nurses, ministers, and seminary students, serving an economically disadvantaged neighborhood. While he was speaking at Howard Medical School in Washington, DC, members of the audience challenged him to consider promoting church clinics in middle- and upper-class neighborhoods so that the clinics would not acquire the stigma of being a form of health care only for the poor. While searching for support for what he was now calling Wholistic Health Centers, Rev. Westberg met with Dr. Edward Lichter, chair of the Department of Preventative Medicine and Community Health at the University of Illinois College of Medicine. Dr. Lichter gave Rev. Westberg an appointment in his department, and together they secured funding from the W. K. Kellogg Foundation to set up several such health centers in Illinois.

Westberg felt strongly that the church was an optimal setting for care:

> We think better health care can be given in the setting of an institution dedicated to healthful living. The average doctor's office does not have the kind of space we have in churches where there are rooms devoted to youth,

music, meditation and many rooms for continuing education classes and seminars. The intention of churches is to
have an active program of learning for people of all ages.
They want their members to be kept abreast of the latest
thinking concerning one's faith and one's life.

Many medical journal articles say that "the way a person looks at life affects his health." Good health care then
requires a more wholistic approach to the many facets of a
person's being related to his illness or health. Our patients
need to be engaged in many different kinds of health-giving
experiences — particularly in support groups where they
meet people who can enrich their lives, give more meaning
to daily living.

We must learn how to utilize the rich human resources to
be found in every congregation, many of which can be put
to use for the upbuilding of people who are in need of the
extra lift from a fellow human. Our Centers will be more
wholistic to the degree they integrate all of their healing
talent with the community of faith, which is the people of
a worshipping congregation who deep down in their heart
would like to find avenues of expression for the gratitude
they feel to God.[6]

In these experimental settings, which became teaching centers
for many doctors, nurses, and pastors from the United States
and abroad, it became clear that the catalyst in the relationship between faith and health was the nurses. Rev. Westberg
observed that the nurses "seemed to have one foot in the sciences
and thereby were able to bridge the unnecessary gap between
these two very old and esteemed professions."[7] Westberg also
observed that nurses

longed to develop creative new methods of teaching and
of relating to patients. . . . Long before anyone wrote articles on wholeness, wellness, and preventative health care,
nurses were already practicing whole person care, at least
for the few moments they were allowed to escape from
the technical aspects of their work. . . . Now is their chance

to reach thousands of people in the informal setting of an institution that is ready to rethink its role in motivating people toward healthy living.[8]

Indeed, the Western medical model is primarily disease oriented, with health defined as absence of disease. Westberg wrote:

> Too often we take care of ourselves more out of a wish to avoid illness than out of a desire to maintain good health. We believe that as long as we don't get sick, we are healthy. In the Christian tradition, [however], health is seen as an ongoing process [which] gives us the energy and vitality to serve and love others, and thus good health is seen in the context of purpose. It is a liberator. With this Christian perspective, we have a good foundation for health promotion, not just disease prevention.[9]

Rev. Westberg went on to say:

> From a biblical perspective, healing is a part of the process of living. Health is on-going; it is not a state that is reached because there are no symptoms of disease. With this in mind, it seems apparent that healing is an activity that is not reserved strictly for the sick. "Healthy" people need care, too. Healing needs to be an everyday occurrence.[10]

Unfortunately, it was soon clear that the cost of financing clinics in churches was prohibitively expensive for most congregations, so Rev. Westberg adapted the model to rely on nurses whom he now called "parish nurses" who could serve as the bridge between the church and medicine. Parish nurses could expand on what the churches were already doing well in regard to health ministry, namely, education and crisis care.[11] However, it must be noted that new models for congregational clinics are springing up, and I would refer you to the outstanding work of Dr. Scott Morris and others at the Church Health Center in Memphis.[12]

The Birth of Parish Nursing

As a practical argument for health care in the church, Westberg understood the unique communal aspect of the social support the church offered across the lifespan:

> [The church] welcomes people of all ages. It welcomes many family configurations, and our families provide the main health support system for most of us. To have an institution that nourishes such a support system is invaluable. ... The church is a powerful influence in our lives. It is one of the few places where it is acceptable to talk about and examine our values and our life-styles and see whether they are in conflict or in harmony with each other.
>
> In the church we are accepted both in sickness and in health. We don't need a pain for our ticket of admission, yet we are still accepted if we do get sick. One of the great advantages of this relationship is that when we do become ill, we are surrounded by people who have known us in health. They know our strengths even though those strengths may now be hidden because we are consumed by illness. They are able to call forth in us those strengths that can help us overcome our illness.[13]

Westberg felt strongly that nurses were the health professionals who could make this form of health ministry possible. Lutheran General Hospital was committed to financially supporting a pilot parish nurse program and in 1985 began to place parish nurses in congregations around the Chicago metropolitan area. (Lutheran General Hospital merged with Evangelical Health System in 1995 to form Advocate Health Care. Advocate continues to support parish nursing in the Chicago area.)

Lutheran General was also committed to the growth and development of parish nursing elsewhere, and in 1985 they created the Parish Nurse Resource Center (later to become the International Parish Nurse Resource Center, or IPNRC). Under the direction of Phyllis Ann Solari-Twadell, RN, MSN, the IPNRC grew rapidly to provide support for parish nursing in the United

States and abroad. Shortly thereafter, Rev. Westberg and others founded the Health Ministries Association as a membership organization for parish nurses and others interested in health ministry.

In 1986, the Parish Nurse Resource Center sponsored a professional meeting for parish nurses, called the "Westberg Symposium," as a venue for presenting research and practice patterns in parish nursing. Now starting into its third decade, the Westberg Symposium continues as an annual conference that is sponsored by Deaconess Parish Nurse Ministries in St. Louis, where IPNRC has been located since January 2002.

In 1987, Rev. Dr. Westberg and his youngest daughter, Jill Westberg McNamara, wrote their seminal work, *The Parish Nurse: How to Start a Parish Nurse Program in Your Church.*[14] This resource helped others learn about their vision for parish nursing, which was beginning to take shape in Illinois, Iowa, Missouri, Wisconsin, and a few other areas around the Midwest.

Parish nursing in St. Louis began at Deaconess Health System on the occasion of the centennial of the founding of the Evangelical Deaconess Sisterhood by Rev. Richard Ellerbrake, who served for a number of years on the board of managers of Deaconess Parish Nurse Ministries. Rev. Ellerbrake's vision led to what is now the largest network of paid professional parish nurses in the world, located in St. Louis.

The work of Rev. Dr. Westberg, Jill Westberg McNamara, and others in Chicago put a name to what had been a movement of the Holy Spirit under way for quite some time. Nurses had been visiting parishioners in homes since the infancy of nursing. In fact, one can say that the entire nursing profession had been profoundly influenced by parish nursing, given the educational experience of Florence Nightingale at Kaiserswerth, Germany, where the work of nurses as parish deaconesses was held in such high regard.

While Rev. Westberg gave this rebirth of deaconess nursing the moniker "parish nursing," a number of registered nurses, such as Judy Teuscher, a member of the Missouri District of the Lutheran Church Missouri Synod, had been doing what was in essence parish nursing since the 1960s. Teuscher would accompany her husband, who was a pastor, on home visits. She was doing health assessments and interventions, while integrating faith and health, long before this form of health ministry had a name and was recognized as a specialized nursing practice by the American Nurses Association.

Other nurses, for example, Evangelical Deaconess Sister Bena Fuchs, had been doing this work before the First World War, relating to churches such as those Evangelical churches connected with the Caroline Mission in St. Louis. Her diary is filled with stories of a wholistic approach to health care, including securing health care access, arranging for referrals to other resources, coordinating volunteers, doing health care assessment and intervention — indeed, her work included all the roles of the parish nurse of today.[15] What is very old — in fact reaching back to the parish deaconesses of Kaiserswerth — has become new again.

Currently, approximately five thousand parish nurses have completed the IPNRC's Parish Nurse Basic Preparation course, and a few thousand more nurses have attended other parish nurse classes. Many other registered nurses who have not yet attended such a class are working in health ministry as well. There probably are close to eleven thousand parish nurses in the United States and growing numbers in other countries around the world, including Canada, Korea, Australia, New Zealand, Swaziland, Madagascar, Zambia, South Africa, Zimbabwe, Ghana, the Bahamas, Singapore, England, Scotland, and Wales. Suffice it to say that parish nursing is growing rapidly. Interest in and research on parish nursing is exploding.

Theological Grounding for Parish Nursing and Health Ministries

Granger Westberg believed that the church was called to "preach, teach, *and* heal." He wrote:

> When Christ sent the disciples out, he didn't just say, "Go out and preach and preach." He said, "Go preach and

heal." Go preach the Kingdom of God and heal the sick.
His own ministry was so integrated. He never dealt with a
body apart from the person's spirit. But he also never dealt
with the spirit apart from the body. He was always dealing
with whole people; I believe that perhaps we in the church
have been remiss in that we have turned the body over to
the scientists, and we have said, "You take care of the body,
and we'll take care of the spirit" — as if you could separate
the two. You cannot separate the body and the spirit; so
it looks as if the scientist and the theologian are going to
have to get back together again.[16]

Westberg found healing central in God's agenda of caring for
suffering humanity:

Theologian Krister Stendahl has written, "God's agenda is
the mending of creation." Mending is an expression for
God's total love toward suffering humanity, of which healing is one aspect.... The rhythm of preaching, teaching,
and healing runs all through Christ's ministry.... All of life
is interrelated and tied to health. The individual human
being is an integrated totality of body, mind, and spirit. The
health of a human being is affected by the various conditions and influences that are a part of life. Jesus understood
this, and in Hebrew culture the body and spirit were not
divorced. Jesus viewed the individual as an essential unit,
and because of this he was able to envision the essential
wholeness of life. Though he was always concerned about
healing a person whose body showed signs of physical illness, he rarely stopped there. He paid close attention as
well to other manifestations of brokenness in that person's
life.[17]

Westberg also was deeply disturbed by the depersonalizing and
fragmented type of health care that hospitals — most started by
the churches — were offering, and he found hope in the type
of healing ministry that parish nurses had to offer, reframing a
theological insight of Martin Buber:

Science, by its very nature, has always tended to have an "I-it" relationship to whatever is being studied. The scientist in the laboratory observes an object that can be manipulated or measured or weighed. The scientist is the "I" dealing with the "it." And this is quite proper. But when the science is the practice of medicine, the "I-it" approach should be limited to certain areas such as laboratory research.... Parish nurses seek to bring the "I-thou" dimension to every human contact.[18]

While parish nurses had far less power than physicians and health systems, he saw in their compassion the power of God:

When thoughtful theologians talk about God, they usually say it would be better for us to describe God as being like Christ. The God we know is the God who was revealed to us in Jesus Christ. We would not think to describe Jesus using the same words that we would use to describe a dictator or a person of great power. The words that are appropriate for Jesus are words like loving, understanding, helpful, healing, compassionate, humble, self-sacrificing — these are words that readily come to mind when we think of him. But having said that, we realize that these words do not tell the whole story of his greatness because he was a very powerful man. He changed the face of human history.... Christ attracted people to him because of his loving spirit, because of his understanding nature, because of his willingness to allow people to be themselves — not to preach at them, but to accept them just as they were and to say things like, "Neither do I condemn thee. Go thy way and sin no more." That's the real power of Jesus.[19]

As with any Zeitgeist, others are consumed by similar ideas, and Westberg was in conversation with people such as Michael Wilson, the author of *The Church Is Healing* (a work that challenged the church to reclaim a role in healing along with medicine, and that received wide interest in Great Britain and the United States in the late 1960s).[20] He also maintained a correspondence with Thomas Droege of Valparaiso University (later the first director of the Interfaith Health Program at the Carter Center), who was interested in the "Religious Roots of Wholistic Health Care," penning an important essay under that title that was included in a 1979 work edited by Westberg entitled *Theological Roots of Wholistic Health Care.*[21] A more contemporaneous theologian speaking about parish nursing is Rev. Richard Ellerbrake, who started parish nursing in St. Louis soon after it began in Chicago. Delivering the Helen J. Westberg Lecture at the Sixteenth Annual Westberg Symposium in St. Louis in 2002, Ellerbrake stated that parish nurses were to fulfill a prophetic role, speaking for God's interests to the sick and suffering. He pointed to Micah 6:8, "What does the Lord require of you, but to do justice, and to love mercy, and to walk humbly with your God."

> Today's parish nurses are in the not-for-profit arena. This is too bad, because it implies that profit is none of their concern. For what it's worth (there's a profitable word), the word "profit" occurs thirty-six times in the entire Bible, Old and New Testaments. Change the spelling from "p-r-o-f-i-t" to "p-r-o-p-h-e-t," and the word occurs more than six hundred times.
>
> Clearly, the prophets did not talk very much about profit. Prophecy is gift of the spirit. I don't mean prophecy as in forecasting the future, but I mean prophecy in the Biblical sense, wherein one speaks for God, on behalf of God for the sake of God's children. This means leadership in tough areas of social life. It means intolerance for our abysmal childhood immunization rates; it means seeking bone, tissue, and organ donors, from every possible candidate; it means community leadership in the wise stewardship of resources, and participation in councils where decisions are made that affect the lives of our neighbors.
>
> Speaking for God's interests means continually plumbing the depths to see what direction commitment to service will take us: how do we ease the pain? How do we strengthen

life? How do we reach beyond our walls to the hurting, wherever they may be? What about the responsibility of the powerful to take care of the vulnerable and the poor? The strong can fend for themselves. This is a tall order. To keep a firm grip as you rise to the challenge, remember the woodpecker with its zygodactyl toes, two pointing forward and two pointing backward, great for keeping a grip on slippery, vertical surfaces. Today's prophetic parish nurses are grounded in the faith, walking humbly with God, and also pointed up to the stars as they peck away at the injustices that abound.[22]

The concept of parish nursing that Granger Westberg envisioned was both old and innovative, forging a new path down a road trod by faithful clergy, laity, and health professionals a century earlier. Rev. Westberg gave the parish nursing movement a name and a strong theological underpinning, and he also had the amazing tenacity and vision to see parish nursing take hold throughout the United States and in several other countries before his death at age eighty-five on February 16, 1999. We — clergy, parish nurses, and laity — would do well to follow in his remarkable footsteps to bring the world a little closer to wholeness and build new bridges between the historical partners of hospitals and faith communities.

Indeed, the world is crying out for this kind of healing. In a world that dehumanizes people in so many ways, that wobbles ever nearer to the brink of military destruction and faces huge health challenges such as AIDS, SARS, and avian flu (not to mention the more mundane threats of diseases such as malaria and other health-related crises such as widespread malnutrition), we sorely need the "I-thou" dimension in every human contact. We are part of a world greatly in need of mending. Jill Westberg McNamara recently put it this way:

God worked through Jesus to bring about radical reforms. Reforms in Judaism, reforms in how women and children were treated, reforms in how people with disabilities were

looked upon ... the list goes on and on. And how he ac-
complished these reforms had nothing to do with good
manners. He argued with the rabbis and hung out with
tax collectors. He listened to women.

When Jesus died, God was not done. Throughout centuries, God has worked through some pretty remarkable
people as well as some pretty ordinary people to bring
about changes. And not just changes that Jesus advocated.
There were also new changes. Perhaps changes inspired by
Jesus, but not specifically stated by him.

We need to rock the boat. We need to risk speaking
and acting from the depths of our hearts. We need to
do things a little differently so that we can see improvements in the health of individuals, communities of faith,
and communities at large ... all of the world.[23]

Krister Stendahl, Martin Buber, Florence Nightingale, Granger
Westberg, Jill Westberg McNamara, and others were right about
the nature of God, calling us to healing and wholeness. We know
this as Christians through Jesus — our Savior, our example, and
the author of our faith — because he was a wonderful storyteller.
Many of his stories have come down to us through the centuries.

Granger Westberg laid the groundwork for Wholistic Health
Centers and Parish Nursing. Let us now take a closer look at the
nursing specialty he helped to create.

Notes

1. "A Brief History of the Parish Nurse Program," in Granger E. Westberg and Jill Westberg McNamara, *The Parish Nurse: Providing a Minister
of Health for Your Congregation* (Minneapolis: Augsburg, 1990), 15.

2. Carol Taylor, Carol Lillis, and Priscilla LeMone, *Fundamentals of
Nursing: The Art and Science of Nursing Care,* 4th ed. (Philadelphia:
Lippincott, 2001).

3. Granger E. Westberg, *Granger Westberg Verbatim: A Vision for
Faith and Health,* ed. William M. Peterson (Chicago: Westberg Institute,
1982; quoted from 2nd ed. St. Louis: International Parish Nurse Resource
Center, 2003), 10.

4. "Wholistic and Holistic," in ibid., 43.

5. "A Historical Perspective," in ibid., 47.

6. "Why Wholistic Health Centers Started in Churches," in ibid., 61.

7. Westberg and Westberg McNamara, *The Parish Nurse,* 17.

8. Ibid., 19–20.

9. Ibid., 37–38.

10. Ibid., 76.

11. Ibid., 38–39.

12. More information about the Church Health Center of Memphis can be found at *www.churchhealthcenter.org* or by contacting G. Scott Morris, MD, MDiv (executive director) or Ann W. Langston (director), 1210 Peabody Avenue, Memphis, TN 38104. Telephone: 901-272-7170.

13. Westberg and Westberg McNamara, *The Parish Nurse,* 39.

14. An updated edition of this book was published by Augsburg in 1990, as cited with the revised title in this chapter.

15. Sister Bena Fuchs's handwritten diary is available in the Deaconess Health System archives now housed in the Eden Theological Seminary Library. Used by permission of Ruth Rasche, archivist of the collection until 1997.

16. Westberg, *Granger Westberg Verbatim,* 40.

17. Ibid., 71–72.

18. Ibid., 69–70.

19. "God — All Powerful?" ibid., 87.

20. Michael Wilson, *The Church Is Healing* (London: SCM Press, 1967).

21. Granger E. Westberg, ed., *Theological Roots of Wholistic Health Care* (Hinsdale, IL: Wholistic Health Centers, 1979), 5–47.

22. Helen J. Westberg Lecture delivered by Rev. Richard Ellerbrake, September 2002, Sixteenth Annual Westberg Parish Nurse Symposium, St. Louis.

23. Jill Westberg McNamara, *Health and Wellness: What Your Faith Community Can Do* (Cleveland: Pilgrim Press, 2006), 21.

Called into Health Ministry

Toni Schaefer, RN, BA, Parish Nurse,
Goderich, Ontario, Canada

"Toni, do you believe in the hand of God?" With these words, my journey into parish nursing ministry began....

Working at a children's rehabilitation center, in Sarnia, Ontario, and living alone, I was content and enjoying life. A colleague of mine approached me on June 1, 2004, with the words above, and my comfortable life changed irrevocably.

Colleen had been having coffee with her parents who live in Goderich, Ontario. They were ready to go when her mom asked if she knew someone who could be a parish nurse in Goderich. Colleen said yes, and my life set out on a new course. Immediately, I felt called.

The ministry description was for a parish nurse to work in three faith communities: Knox Presbyterian Church, North Street United Church, and St. Peter's Roman Catholic Church. When I was offered the position, I felt comfortable in quitting my job, selling my house, and never looking back.

I am contracted by the Perth-Huron Victorian Order of Nurses in Stratford, Ontario, who help financially and professionally.

I have office space in each of the three churches and have been contracted for ten hours a week at each church. The three churches view this as outreach/mission and are not jealous of their time allotment. Needs are sometimes greater in one of the churches in a given week, and the others don't mind if I spend more time at one church than the others.

Programs are offered for all churches and usually the community at large. I have had a health fair; a five-part series called "Reasons for Sadness," dealing with the faces of depression; and an ongoing, bi-weekly, and informal women's forum dealing with women's health issues. It is called "What Women Want." There is a team of caring visitors in each church who are trained and supported with debriefing meetings and interdenominational education. Members of the team are encouraged to see me individually with concerns. They are a visible sign that the churches care for their people.

Another branch of Caring Visitors makes "Care Quilts." A member of the United Church asked if I could use quilts to give to people as a tangible gift of the churches' concern for individuals. In one year's time, fifty-eight quilts have been given out, some to as far away as Ottawa. Each quilt bears a label that says, "Wrap Yourself in Love." Then there is a space for the person's name and the words, "A gift from [name of church]."

I am privileged to be accepted into each faith community. I attend all three churches, but not on the same day. I usually make two services almost every Sunday. I have conducted a service at North Street when the ministers have been absent, and given the reflection for Mind, Body, and Spirit Sunday at Knox. I promote wellness in mind, body, and spirit in the call to live our faith fully, both individually and through the "Nurse's Station" in the Sunday bulletins. These educational blurbs also go out to five other church bulletins in the community, as I am part of the ministerial association.

I have a wonderful pastoral care team in one church, an active health council in another, and a supportive minister in the third. I also have a supportive husband. I married Bill Schaefer in November. He was and still is a strong advocate of parish nursing and was instrumental in its inception at Knox Presbyterian Church, in 1998, before it was an interdenominational position. He was one of the panel that interviewed me for the position. Who would have thunk?

I look forward to almost every day as a parish nurse. I treasure the fact that it is interdenominational and I have grown because of that aspect. It may be a drop in the bucket, but that drop is better than what they had before, and all appreciate what they do have. The Spirit of God is always being called upon in my ministry to help me find the words or do the right thing. My motto is "I do my best and God does the rest." I also know that I came to tend, but I was the one tended.

Two

Parish Nursing

A Beneficial Partnership for Clergy

Parish nurses are often thought of as nice older ladies who stand around during coffee hour, measuring blood pressure with one hand and giving flu shots with the other. Let me dispel some myths:

Myth #1: Parish nurses are nice older ladies. Well, they generally are older, and nice. But many parish nurses are in their thirties, and the rest forty or older. What they all have in common, however, is a wealth of experience in health care, from hospital settings to home health, from pediatrics to gerontology, from oncology to AIDS research. Growing numbers of parish nurses are men, as well.

Myth #2: Parish nurses work only with the people within the congregation. Well, they do work with the people in the congregation they serve, but depending on the size of the church, they generally end up spending a great deal of time working with the neighbors in the surrounding area (the traditional idea of "parish"). That is why we have stuck with the term "parish nurse," because we want to encourage outreach to the broader community.

Here are some of the ways that parish nurses reach out into the community:

• A week after Hurricane Frances hit the eastern coast of Florida, Interfaith Health and Wellness Association (IHWA) received a phone call to help a Red Cross shelter in Paho-kee. Within three hours, parish nurses were able to coordinate same-day delivery of a truckload of supplies: diapers, for-mula, water, and personal items from the area distribution center of the United Methodist Churches in West Palm Beach; collection of personal items by school children and their fam-ilies from St. Paul's Lutheran Church and School in Boca Raton; and collection of flood items and insect repellent by children and their families from St. Jude Catholic Church in Boca Raton.

• Mary Ann Brischetto, RN, BSN, parish nurse at St. Paul United Church of Christ in St. Louis, has worked with more than two hundred families at risk of falling apart due to severe economic and emotional challenges. Most of those families have been successful in building healthy lives, and there is a waiting list to get into her parenting program, which serves the broader St. Louis community.

• Nancy Moore, RN, parish nurse at Tucker Swamp Baptist Church in Zuni, Virginia, has developed an outreach program for people who, because of disease or disability, are unable to care for their feet. "Sole Care" takes place once a month at the church, with the community invited. Nancy publicizes this outreach program in the local newspapers and on the local radio stations in their free broadcast times.

• Nancy Merila, RN, parish nurse at Mount Calvary Lutheran Church, Brentwood, Missouri, is known as "Nurse Nancy" in the health education column she writes for the local newspaper and on a show she does for a local cable network.

• Elizabeth Durban, RN, parish nurse at St. Gabriel Catho-lic Church, St. Louis, hosts health fairs that regularly attract hundreds of local residents from the community through at-tractions such as seeing the inside of an ambulance, great food, engaging speakers, and a very well organized and well publicized event.

Myth #3: About those blood pressure screenings and flu
shots: parish nurses do screen for hypertension, but invasive screenings (such as a finger prick for cholesterol
or blood sugar) or invasive health care service (such as
flu shots) must be arranged through another health care
provider, such as the Visiting Nurses Association.

And this is just the tip of the iceberg! Let's take a closer look at
this form of health ministry.

What Is Parish Nursing?

Parish nursing is the intentional integration of the practice of
faith with the practice of nursing so that people can achieve
wholeness in, with, and through the community of faith in
which parish nurses serve.[1] Parish nurses educate, advocate, and
activate people to take positive action regarding wellness, prevention, appropriate treatment of illness, and social and spiritual
connections with God, members of their congregations, and their
wider community.

A parish nurse serves a number of roles in a local congregation
and neighborhood. To understand these roles, it is helpful first
to note what a parish nurse is *not:*

+ A parish nurse is not a physician and will not diagnose or
  treat illness.

+ A parish nurse is not a home health care nurse and will not
  dispense medications or provide treatments prescribed by a
  physician.

+ A parish nurse is not a therapist and will not do physical
  therapy, occupational therapy, or psychotherapy.

+ A parish nurse is not a clergyperson. All parish nurses,
  however, come to the field with a deep spiritual commitment.

The roles of a parish nurse usually include the following:

- *Integrator of Faith and Health.* Health is a wholistic way of living that embraces life in its fullness, including the pursuit of a healthy spiritual life and connection to God and God's people. A parish nurse assists parishioners to achieve higher levels of wellness by improving both their spiritual and physical health.

- *Health Educator.* Most physicians have only a few minutes to spend with each of their many patients. Parish nurses are available for health education and provide opportunities to learn about health issues, individually and in groups.

- *Health Counselor.* Parishioners may already have been to physicians but do not fully understand their diagnoses or options for treatment. They may have medications that have been improperly dispensed. They may wonder if their concerns even warrant seeing a doctor. A parish nurse is available to discuss health concerns, emphasizing early response to small problems and encouraging healthy lifestyles.

- *Referral Advisor.* Where does a parishioner go for a second opinion, a good nursing home for a loved one, a counselor, or another service? A parish nurse is available to provide referrals to health care and social services within the community upon request.

- *Health Advocate.* Far too often, patients lose their way in the jagged pieces of the health care system. A parish nurse can help navigate. A parish nurse speaks out to help obtain needed health-related services.

- *Developer of Support Groups.* A community often has need for support groups such as grief support, weight loss support, or caregivers support. A parish nurse facilitates the development of support groups for the faith community and others served.

- *Volunteer Coordinator.* Transportation to medical appointments, food during convalescence, or childcare support can be provided through volunteers. A parish nurse recruits, prepares, and oversees congregational volunteers who help those in need.

A parish nurse's specific assignments within the ministry of a congregation are decided in consultation with other church leaders and/or a "health cabinet" in the parish. They may design an outreach ministry to the surrounding neighborhood, or a very specialized ministry, such as within a school. Most parishes, however, prefer that the parish nurse serves broadly in response to the varied needs of the congregation and neighborhood.

Why Does a Pastor Benefit from Having a Parish Nurse on Staff?

Parish nursing is rewarding work for those registered nurses who are attracted to the field. Parish nursing provides a setting in which to help people regardless of their ability to pay, the opportunity to visit people in the context of their community setting in order to best assess their support networks, and an ability to integrate faith as a factor when doing health assessments and education. However, clergy as well have a great deal to gain from developing parish nursing as part of their congregation's ministry. Here are six reasons that a pastor benefits from having a parish nurse on staff:

1. *Much of a pastor's ministry is health-related.* Pastors deal with parishioner's health concerns on a daily basis — visiting parishioners who are hospitalized, homebound, or residents of nursing homes, for example. Many of the concerns brought to pastors during worship or pastoral care have health-related components. Clergy work daily for the health and wholeness of their congregations. A parish nurse can help support these efforts.

2. *Volunteers are not as available as they were in the past.* The days of having large numbers of church volunteers are over in most places. The pastor is expected to do much of the

work of the church alone. A parish nurse can help share visitation. She or he can also work with a "health cabinet" to identify, train, and support those volunteers who are available, so that their efforts can be coordinated.

3. *Other sectors of the society are looking to churches to pick up the pieces.* Congregations are often called by hospitals to help arrange for supportive care for patients about to be discharged. People are falling through the cracks of the health care system. President Bush's "Faith-Based Initiative" presupposes that churches are able to take on a larger share of care for those in need of assistance, and individuals are coming to congregations for help. Parish nurses can help triage these needs and address those that can be met.

4. *Clergy and the church have leadership roles in health care.* Historically, clergy and the church have played leadership roles in health care, establishing many of the hospitals, for example. It is time for clergy and congregations to reclaim a voice in the health of the community. The parish nursing model is one way to do this and so build a strong bridge between medical and faith communities. A parish nurse understands both worlds well and can help parishioners traverse that divide.

5. *The church has a biblical mandate to "Preach, Teach, and Heal."* As mentioned in chapter 1, if you visit most congregations you will find preaching every week. You will also find teaching most weeks through Sunday School or Adult Education. You might be hard-pressed to find an organized ministry of healing, however. This is a broken and wounded world, and the church is called to follow Jesus in the ministry of healing. Pastors and parish nurses together can do great things in Jesus' name!

6. *Parish nurses improve the health of pastors.* Parish nurses not only advocate for the health of parishioners; they also improve clergy health. The most common changes in health behaviors among congregants with a parish nurse are healthier diets, increased exercise, increased use of seat belts, and

more regular health screenings. Many pastors have improved health (or even their life saved!) thanks to a parish nurse.

The Bottom Line

The bottom line is that parish nursing can be a part of a congregation's ministry that addresses the church's mandate to preach, teach, and heal. It does so in a way that addresses the brokenness in today's health care system (which was started by the church) and in a way that makes the pastor's life easier (and improves the pastor's health too!).

Notes

1. This mission statement for parish nursing was developed by over six hundred parish nurses at the Fourteenth Annual Westberg Symposium in 2000.

HEALTH MINISTRY IN ACTION
A Role Model for the Church

Juanita Jordon, BSN, RN, and Rev. Lorenzo B. Hill Sr.,
John Mann United Methodist Church, Winchester, Virginia

Juanita Jordon began her practice as parish nurse for John Mann United Methodist Church in Winchester, Virginia, in 1997 after completing the IPNEP program in an a RN-BSN class at Shenandoah University. She says that the ministry began as she set up her practice at the church as part of her community clinical experience. She was able to lay a foundation that was solid and gain the approval and confidence of her pastor, Rev. Lorenzo B. Hill Sr. The response was slow at first but has built over the years to very active ministry with many congregants utilizing her knowledge, support, and guidance.

Rev. Hill believed that he needed to be a role model for his congregation, so he began to take the health counseling and teaching that Juanita offered and apply it to his own life. He had marvelous results, and his enthusiasm about his own health improvements began to spill over into the congregation. Rev. Hill has Juanita give a short health tip and teaching topic at the end of each of his sermons as well as at the end of Bible studies.

Since her congregation is mostly African American, Juanita emphasizes education on blood pressure, obesity, and diabetes. She offers blood pressure screenings every Sunday. She accompanies parishioners to the ER and to doctor's appointments. She visits them in the hospital and in their homes. She has a bulletin board with health-related tips and a monthly newsletter. As part of her community outreach, she joins with another parish nurse at a neighboring church for a children's health fair in the spring and an adult health fair in the fall. Attendance averages about three hundred for each fair. Amazingly, she does all this in only eight hours a week.

Juanita says that she has grown spiritually in this ministry in a way she would never have expected. When asked if she had a tip for other parish nurses, she responded quickly: "Pray before you do anything. Stay filled, and take time to listen to the Lord."

Three

The Head Bone's
Connected to the Heart
Parish Nurses as Teachers
in the Congregation

"The head bone's connected to the neck bone." That was about the extent of my medical training as a pastor, and about the extent of the health education I was qualified to teach in the congregations I served. Yet the church is called to "preach, teach, and heal." How are we as clergy and congregations doing with each of those? The church must also integrate these activities: preaching must be more than sermons, teaching must be more than Sunday School, healing must be more than calling 911 if someone faints.

Each member of a church leadership team can play an important part in this integration. Parish nurses, a relatively new addition to the staff of many congregations, can bring health wisdom to share with parishioners and the neighborhood. They know which bone is connected to the next. They also know that health is wholistic. Each part of the body is connected to the heart. Each part of the body is connected to the spirit.

In the context of a faith community, parish nurses have different opportunities to participate in teaching. There is a wide variety of settings in which teaching by parish nurses can occur in a congregation.

Classes Offered for Groups

At first glance, the most obvious place for parish nurses to teach is through classes on health-related topics, and indeed, such offerings abound. During the past year, the parish nurses who are members of the Deaconess Parish Nurse Ministries Network led or sponsored over 130 presentations on topics such as CPR, First Aid, Parenting, Nutrition, Advanced Directives, Heart Health, Bike Safety, West Nile Virus, Stress Management, Mental Health, Emergency Preparedness, Healthy Aging, and Organ Donation, among many others. These presentations were sometimes offered as "stand-alone" classes, but often were part of other events, such as Women's Fellowship meetings or Vacation Bible School programming.

Like any other form of Christian education, however, health ministry education is often most powerfully communicated by way of personal example. The parish nurse needs to be aware that people are watching her to see if she practices what she preaches. (Currently, most parish nurses are women, but there are growing numbers of outstanding parish nurses who are men.) The congregation will be watching to see if the parish nurse exercises, gets enough sleep, drinks water instead of soda, takes a vacation each year, and eats nutritious food. If she doesn't model taking good care of her own health, the parish nurse is unlikely to convince many others to change their personal health practices, no matter how many classes she offers.

One-on-One Teaching

Of course, parish nurses spend a significant amount of time one-on-one with individuals who have concerns about their health and need help gathering further information. Parish nurses reinforce the health education provided by physicians and other health professionals. They are able to do so without the time constraints placed on other health professionals by insurers.

Let me share an example of where a parish nurse, through one-on-one teaching, could have made a difference in preventing an adverse situation for an elderly parishioner. Recently, a woman in a congregation near our office received a pacemaker. She was visited by the physician before her discharge from the hospital, and he went over her instructions. She did not fully understand them, however, and did not realize that she would no longer need to take the same medications she was taking before the procedure. She continued to take those medications, along with her new prescriptions, and became seriously ill after returning home. A parish nurse would have been able to visit the woman immediately upon her return home to be sure that she understood her new treatment protocol. With the parishioner's permission, the parish nurse could have even been with the woman when she met with the physician while she was still in the hospital, or accompanied the woman on a visit to the doctor.[1]

Teaching Moments for the Congregation

Some of the opportunities for health education are aimed at the entire congregation. Here are some opportunities for health education in a congregational setting:

- *A mission moment.* Activities of the health ministry can be shared through a "Mission Moment" in the worship service. Remind people about upcoming health fairs, blood drives, and exercise programs. Make it appealing!

- *Inserts in the bulletin.* This is a good place to publicize your health ministry events, or to share brief health notes of interest. Good sources of health notes can be found online through sources such as the Mayo Clinic's health information website at *www.MayoClinic.com* or the website for children and their parents sponsored by the Nemours Foundation: *www.kidshealth.org.*

- *Articles in the newsletter.* A recent survey we did of parishioners in over one hundred churches with parish nurses found that the overwhelming majority read the articles by parish nurses in their church newsletters. Wonderful resources for materials to include can be found through free or inexpensive health newsletters such as the National Women's Health Resource Center "Health Report," the Johns Hopkins Medical

Letter, the University of California at Berkeley Wellness Letter, and the Nutrition Action Healthletter of the Center for Science in the Public Interest.

* *The bulletin board.* A bulletin board is a great place to highlight national health observances. They are easily found online through the National Health Information Center at *www.healthfinder.gov/library/nho/nho.asp.* Hang lots of colorful photos of people participating in fun health events, such as a Healthy Foods Potluck or a Walking Club. Use this space to inform people of current health issues in their area and if they can take action to help, such as writing a legislator.

* *Brochure rack.* Care Notes from Abbey Press are a great resource. Also, many other organizations will provide free materials for you. Try the American Heart Association, the American Lung Association, and the American Diabetes Association, for example. Many of these organizations have materials specially designed for children that might be suitable for use in Sunday School, children's bulletins, or worship hour packets.

The suggestions listed here are simply examples. There are many other settings for teaching by parish nurses to take place. But I would urge clergy not to discount the important role that they themselves play in teaching and healing during the preaching moment. A recent study by the Health Task Force of the National Council of Churches found that sermons related to health ministry were a critical teaching moment for the congregation.[2] While this is in no way an encouragement to turn the sermon into a "medical minute," it is an encouragement to offer permission to the congregation to discuss challenging issues in sickness and in health.

Notes

1. The HIPAA regulations (Health Insurance Portability and Accountability Act) do allow patients to be accompanied for health services if they

give their permission. We require parish nurses to obtain this permission in writing before accompanying parishioners in this way.

2. The "Congregational Health Ministry Survey Report" of the NCC conducted by Rev. Eileen W. Lindner, PhD, and Rev. Marcel A. Welty. It can be accessed online at *www.health-ministries.org*.

Working with Non-English-Speaking Families

Pat Scott, RN, BSN, Parish Nurse,
First Congregational United Church of Christ,
Janesville, Wisconsin

Wilson Elementary School, located in the same downtown neighborhood as the First Congregational United Church of Christ, is designated as one of three English-Language Learning elementary schools in Janesville, Wisconsin, about an hour south of Madison. In the spring of 2001, the church learned that non-English-speaking parents (primarily Hispanic) were concerned because most of their information about school and activities came from their children and wasn't always accurate. Working with the Parish Care Committee, Pat hosted a number of "Family Gatherings." The first began with supper provided by the church. Now they are potluck, and all bring food to share. Interpreters are provided by the school. Speakers have covered topics such as summer programs for children, city bus service, English classes available, and information on nutrition, immunizations, and other services available through the county. A huge benefit is that families are getting to know each other and feel less isolated.

Approximately forty-five to fifty-five family members plus school staff and members of the Parish Care Committee attended each quarterly gathering last year. In addition, the program has begun creating a series of short videos to reach the Cambodian community, many of whom are not literate. Now after the potluck, the group divides into two groups, and there are educational materials available to both. Through this mission outreach, the parish nurse and the Parish Care Committee are extending a hand of welcome to those new to this country.

Four

You've Seen One Health Ministry, You've Seen One Health Ministry

Outreach on Behalf of the Congregation

At the International Parish Nurse Resource Center we are often asked if parish nurses should work primarily with the congregation or with the community. We answer facetiously, but honestly, "yes!" For the fact is that parish nurses usually develop a balance between the two. Congregations who want a parish nurse to meet the needs of congregants often identify neighbors who also need assistance, and most parish nurses are glad to oblige. Churches who want a parish nurse to address community needs often have congregational members who seek out the parish nurse for health counseling or for information about community health resources. What this looks like as a practical matter generally depends upon the needs and plans of the congregation. Each parish nurse ministry evolves into a unique response to congregational and community health needs, as do all forms of health ministry.

Consider Gayle Mason and Josephine Fields, for example. They are parish nurses who have worked for Union Avenue Christian Church and the United Church Neighborhood Houses, respectively, in a changing urban core neighborhood of St. Louis. A few years ago, Josephine and Gayle discovered that children were "dumpster-diving" after school, going through area dumpsters, and they noticed it was a pattern. Upon investigation, they found the children were searching for food. In a school where 99 percent of the children were living in poverty, the children were hungry and faced the prospect of remaining hungry until the next school day. The nurses worked with the administration at the school and with a local food bank to arrange for a "Kids Café" to provide a meal for the children after school, so that, combined with their school breakfast and lunch, they would have three meals a day.

Parish Nursing as Outreach

Parish nurse ministry can focus on outreach to the community through each of the following roles. Most of the work that a parish nurse does, however, is done in conjunction with a health cabinet.

*   *Integrator of Faith and Health.* The parish nurse might offer classes to the community, in conjunction with the pastor, on topics such as "The Bible and Wellness," "Spiritual Resources for Coping with Chronic Illness," or "Prayer and the Caregiver." The possibilities for topics that integrate faith and health are limitless.

*   *Health Educator.* Many health education programs offered by congregations are open to the public or are made available to area schools, such as a "Hip Hop for a Healthy Heart" event that was held by a parish nurse who does a great deal of work with children in her neighborhood. Held as an afterschool program on a Monday evening, it stared at 4:30 p.m. (after the kids had done their homework), and included several choices of healthy snacks.

*   *Health Counselor.* Some congregations offer outreach to neighbors through such ministries as food pantries, soup kitchens, or emergency assistance. Often a parish nurse is able to help people with health concerns who come to the church for these services. In other cases, parishioners ask if the parish nurse would be willing to meet with a neighbor who has health questions.

◆ *Referral Advisor.* People from the community who come to the pastor for help often have health-related questions. The parish nurse can be available to help with referral to appropriate agencies for help, particularly in emergency situations.

◆ *Health Advocate.* The parish nurse can help educate parishioners on topics such as changes in Medicare coverage, and the classes that she or he offers on these topics can be made available to all. Parish nurses are also generally willing to meet with individuals in their homes to discuss such matters and are glad to meet with friends or neighbors of parishioners.

◆ *Developer of Support Groups.* Some people (author included) need peer pressure to get moving. Regular exercise is an important component of promoting good health. A parish nurse could organize a walking group in the church gymnasium and open it to the community. He or she could also arrange for classes such as karate to be taught for a modest fee to neighborhood children. Funding for this type of program can often be found through local foundations or businesses, especially when they know that the programs are open to all in the community. This type of outreach is a way to reclaim the integration of body, mind, spirit, *and* community.

◆ *Volunteer Coordinator.* A parish nurse who coordinates volunteers can "multiply the ministry" of a congregation. Barbara Sage, for example, the director of the Nurse and Health Ministries Network at Beatitudes Center DOAR (Developing Older Adult Resources) in Phoenix, worked with forty to fifty volunteers at Orangewood Nazarene Church. They did hospital and home visitation, took other parishioners to medical visits, prepared meals for those recuperating at home following a hospitalization, and had a card ministry to those who were home-based. She met with the volunteers after church on a monthly basis for support, networking, and training on how to make hospital visits and to share resources, for example, as information about what was available in the durable medical equipment closet.

Hairdressers, Gardens, and Fairs

As you can see, parish nurses can participate in significant outreach on behalf of congregations. Here are some other ideas that have worked for a number of our parish nurses:

- Offer to write a health column for your local newspaper, especially if you live in a smaller town or have a paper for your suburb or neighborhood. Some of the parish nurses have even appeared on TV.

- Organize a Health Fair for the beginning of the school year for the families in your community. You might be able to find someone who will give haircuts and school supplies. Invite health providers who will provide vision, hearing, and other screenings free of charge (sometimes fire departments will provide screenings). Be sure you advertise it widely, and offer a "draw" to the event. Do you have free lunch? Do you have prizes? What are the "take-aways" to entice the community to walk through your doors?[1]

- Start a Community Garden. This is a great way to educate neighborhood children about nutrition and teach them about the joys of growing their own food. One parish nurse includes field trips to the local farmers' market.

- Reach out to beauty shop and barber shop owners in the neighborhood to educate them on the warning signs for stroke, which can often be treated if recognized quickly. People are often willing to tell their hairdresser how they feel, and only 2 percent of the population knows the warning signs of a stroke. By the way, these are the warning signs of a stroke:

  - Sudden numbness or weakness of the face, arm, or leg, especially on one side of the body
  - Sudden confusion, trouble speaking or understanding
  - Sudden trouble seeing in one or both eyes
  - Sudden trouble walking, dizziness, loss of balance or coordination
  - Sudden, severe headache with no known cause.

Call 911 if you or someone else is experiencing any or all of these symptoms. Appropriate medication given within three hours of the onset of symptoms can prevent or reduce disability from a stroke.[2]

- Make friends with the postal delivery staff and have them be on the lookout for people who might need health assistance.

- Educate about health at community events. For example, on the Fourth of July, parades go by many churches in America. Why not pass out bottled water with flyers explaining the importance of drinking six to eight glasses of water a day?

- Many parish nurses make their services available to the families who use the day-care centers in their churches. They can also give classes for the day-care teachers about safety, hygiene, and first aid, to name just a few.

Notes

1. For a good article on putting together a health cabinet, see Elizabeth Durbin (parish nurse at St. Gabriel's Catholic Church, St. Louis) in *The Essential Parish Nurse: ABCs for Congregational Health Ministry* (Cleveland: Pilgrim Press, 2004).

2. Information from the American Heart Association.

Parish Nursing "Outside the Box"

Parish nursing, or faith community nursing, has been moving "outside the box." Deaconess Parish Nurse Ministries (DPNM) in St. Louis currently employs parish nurses in several dozen congregations, but also supports parish nurses working in several faith-based organizations and is exploring other possibilities. Here are a few observations on their work.

First of all, it is important to note that the parish nurses working in these non-traditional sites are extremely motivated and self-directed. They are incredible! U'Essie Riley is a parish nurse for a day-care center in a very blighted neighborhood of East St. Louis, where the poverty level approaches that of any third-world country. She also coordinates health services/education efforts for an after-school program at the Christian Activity Center nearby. Linda Spina works with Nurses for Newborns, providing services to fragile families with children under the age of two. Ann Sutherlin is a parish nurse working in a faith-based senior living center.

Patricia Townes was recently featured in the Mid-America Transplant Services (MTS) 2006 annual report under the headline "A National First." Pat works with St. John's Community Ministry and with Isaiah 58, two church-based social service organizations that provide food, clothing, and other support. Her parish nursing practice is unique in that it is funded through MTS to help reduce the incidence of diseases leading to the need for organ transplantation.

Joyce Gusewelle Lony serves as both a parish nurse and the director of the Interfaith Volunteer Caregivers program at Eden United Church of Christ in Edwardsville, Illinois, providing free transportation, meals, housekeeping, and other home-based support to seniors and disabled individuals needing extra support to remain in their homes.

Altogether, the parish nurses at Deaconess Parish Nurse Ministries are overseeing a total of approximately 150 programs to promote the health and well-being of the congregations and area neighborhoods.

DPNM usually has been able to locate grant funding to get parish nurses started, covering part of the parish nurse salary for the first two or three years, as an organization moves toward paying the full amount of salary for the parish nurse. Rarely can an organization pay the full parish nurse salary in the first year.

All the parish nurses named above are paid, and only rarely have the organizations been unable to pick up their increasing share of the salary. In those cases, DPNM helped to raise funds to cover the difference and has never had to close any organizational parish nurse program. Some have been going for over a decade.

All the parish nurses work at least ten hours a week in each setting. Some combine parish work with organizational work. For example, Ann Sutherlin works ten hours a week at Holy Name of Jesus Parish and ten hours a week for Cape Albeon Senior Retirement Living. Others, like Rev. Fields, work full time as a parish nurse.

The Spirit of the Lord is bringing healing and wholeness in so many ways. We are thrilled to be able to partner with other organizations to provide parish nursing in this unique way.

Five

In Sickness and in Health

Health and Wholeness for Adults

Within the Judeo-Christian tradition (and in most other faiths as well), we believe and claim that we are not alone. "I have called you by name, you are mine," says the Lord (Isaiah 43:1).

As the church, we are one Body in Christ, and we need to care about one another — in sickness *and* in health. We can coax one another into changing health behaviors: exercising more regularly, eating more healthful food. We can help one another get to the doctor and navigate our way through the increasingly complex health care system, both the system of care, and the system of paying for that care. We can arm ourselves with knowledge shared by others, such as doctors and other health educators.

Rev. Dr. Granger Westberg wrote, "Health is not a solitary endeavor. That is why the Hebrew Scriptures are filled with health laws for the community to observe together. That is why we have exercise clubs, YMCAs, and track teams. That is why we have support groups to help each other lose weight, stop smoking, and keep moving."[1]

A conference held recently in Chapel Hill, North Carolina, called "The Power of Connection: Group Health Care for the 21st Century," provided further evidence for effectiveness of the group model of health promotion. Data presented there showed that using this model with prenatal care was able to reduce the level of preterm delivery by *a third,* a remarkable result involving two simple changes: group support and the opportunity to spend more time with health providers, such as nurses.[2]

Adult men and women share similar risk for many health issues. According to the latest statistics from the National Center for Health Statistics at the Centers for Disease Control and Prevention (CDC), heart disease continues to be the leading cause of death for men and women, with more than 650,000 people succumbing to this disease each year. Cancer is a close second, accounting for approximately half a million deaths a year. Stroke, respiratory disease, accidents (unintentional injuries), diabetes, and Alzheimer's disease follow in rank order. Flu and pneumonia account for more than 60,000 deaths a year, with nephritis and septicemia completing the "Top 10" list.

It should be noted, however, that men (particularly those in the twenty-one-to-sixty-five-year-old age group) are often reluctant to schedule medical appointments for routine checkups or what they perceive are minor health concerns. Women may falsely believe their gender to keep them at much lower risk of heart disease. A health ministry team can help to support wellness and early intervention for illness detection and treatment.

Sadly, however, in the richest country in the world, many adults have a difficult time accessing a primary care physician to help with tracking their health concerns. The American College of Physicians, representing U.S. internists, recently released a report, "The Impending Collapse of Primary Care Medicine and Its Implications for the State of the Nation's Health Care." The title sounds ominous, but here are the facts they present:

- Forty-five percent of the United States population has a chronic medical condition, and about half (of 60 million people) have more than one chronic condition.[3]

- Eighty-three percent of individuals over age sixty-five have multiple chronic conditions and nearly one-quarter of that group (23 percent) has five or more chronic conditions.[4] By 2030, one-fifth of the U.S. population will be over the age of sixty-five.[5]

- Thirty-five percent of U.S. physicians are over age fifty-five and will retire in the next five to ten years.[6]

- In 1998, 57 percent of third-year internal medical residents were entering primary care, but that number had dropped to 19 percent by 2003.[7]

- "When compared with other developed countries, the United States ranked lowest in its primary care functions and lowest in health care outcomes, yet highest in health care spending."[8]

The report urged reforms to the payment structures that reward performing procedures, such as heart transplants, but provide few incentives for prevention. While we wait for reform, what can be done?

Parish nurses are a "friend in health care" who can help people of all ages understand their health conditions and medications, navigate the health system, and follow their treatment protocols. Here are some of the ways that parish nurses have helped adults in congregations in a variety of settings:

- *Exercise programs.* "Walk to Jerusalem ... " is a church-based walking program that encourages participants to track the numbers of miles they walk (or the time they swim or otherwise exercise at the equivalent of twenty minutes per mile). Then they add their total during Lent to those of other participants in the church with the goal of walking the number of miles from their congregation's location to Jerusalem. Cathy White at St. Margaret of Scotland in St. Louis had over 150 people sign up the first week! They took a lot of "side tours" on their way to Jerusalem. For more information about this program, visit the website of St. John Health (a health system based in Michigan) at *www.stjohn.org/WalktoJerusalem/*.

- *"Brown Bag Day."* This is a "triple whammy" health education event, scheduled three times over the summer after worship services by the Health and Wellness Committee led by parish nurse Nancy Merila at Mount Calvary Lutheran Church in Brentwood, Missouri. Parishioners were invited to bring their medications (in a brown bag for privacy) for review by clinical pharmacy students, under the supervision of a faculty member. The pharmacy students discussed potential drug interactions or concerns with parishioners. A freewill offering was taken to help send a medical team to South Africa. A second aspect of "Brown Bag Day" was the "Brown Bag Lunch" served by the youth group, which was raising money to prepare for their mission trip to Mexico to build houses. The lunches were healthy sandwiches, veggies, and a small home-baked cookie. The final treat for the day was "A Healthy Taste," which gave parishioners samples of three or four different items that were healthy, easy to prepare, and tasty. The recipes were chosen and pretested by the Health and Wellness Committee, and recipes were shared with all the parishioners. Even kids asked for the recipes, so that their parents could make the healthy foods!

- *Oral health.* The American Heart Association points to research done at Boston University and Harvard University showing that poor oral health is associated with coronary heart disease. Busy adults (particularly men) often neglect their oral health. Parish nurses in St. Louis have arranged for faculty from the dental schools to make presentations at area congregations.

- *Mental health counseling.* A number of parish nurses have worked with local counseling agencies to provide counselors to congregations on a sliding-scale basis. Often it works well to collaborate with other area congregations, so parishioners can visit a counselor in a more private location.

- *Weight loss programs.* Parish nurses offer a number of programs encouraging healthy weight and balancing healthy eating, exercise, and group support. Programs they have used include "Weigh Down" and "3–D." A good recent resource is *Fat-Proof Your Family,* by J. Ron Eaker, MD, published by Bethany House.

- *"Health Minutes."* Some parish nurses have accepted offers from parishioners to speak about health issues that have affected them during a "Health Minute" during a worship service or coffee hour. Having someone willing to talk from the heart about cancer or diabetes can help others struggling with similar concerns.

◆ *Bulletin and newsletter materials.* Most parish nurses create "bulletin blurbs" and newsletter articles on health issues as a regular feature. Some have even taken their articles to local papers and TV stations.

◆ *Help with navigating the health care system.* A number of parish nurses have invited "ombudsmen" or other helping professionals to talk with parishioners about navigating their way through the maze of health care resources and financing mechanisms. There are many different ways that health insurance works, and often we find out only "after the fact" what could have been done.

◆ *Help in accessing care.* With 47 million uninsured (and many more underinsured) in this country, parish nurses often spend a great deal of time helping people find access to care, either through doctors willing to accept private pay patients, through negotiating discounted rates on behalf of parishioners, or through locating other public sources of care. Many congregations are also active in efforts such as "Cover the Uninsured Week," an initiative of the Robert Wood Johnson Foundation working to provide health care coverage for all.

◆ *Smoking cessation.* Churches have long worked with organizations such as Alcoholics Anonymous to help folks struggling with alcoholism. Less easy to find are programs in congregations that help people stop smoking. Programs aimed at helping people quit smoking (and keeping kids from starting) are springing up around the country. For more information, contact the Campaign for Tobacco-Free Kids, which has a number of faith-based initiatives (*www.tobaccofreekids.org*).

Parish nurses provide "womb to tomb" care and support — including prenatal classes for expectant mothers, child safety classes, adolescent health programs, adult exercise promotion, and support for the isolated elderly.

Notes

1. "Westberg as a Patient," in *Granger Westberg Verbatim* (St. Louis: International Parish Nurse Resource Center, 2003), 55.

2. Peter S. Bernstein, MD, MPH, "Care of Patients in Groups: The New Model of Healthcare," *www.medscape.com/viewarticle/529462?src=mp*, accessed May 19, 2006.

3. Shin-Yi Wu and Anthony Green, "Projection of Chronic Illness Prevalence and Cost Inflation," Santa Monica, CA: RAND Corporation (October 2000).

4. G. F. Anderson, "Medicare and Chronic Conditions," Sounding Board, *New England Journal of Medicine* 353, no. 3 (2005): 305–9.

5. Wu and Green, "Projection of Chronic Illness Prevalence and Cost Inflation."

6. Physician Characteristics and Distribution in the United States. American Medical Association data, 2005.

7. R. N. Garibaldi, C. Popkave, and W. Bylsma, "Career Plans for Trainees in Internal Medicine Residency Programs," *Academic Medicine* 80 (2005): 507–12.

8. "The Impending Collapse of Primary Care Medicine and Its Implications for the State of the Nation's Health Care," a Report from the American College of Physicians, January 30, 2006. Studies quoted are the following: B. Starfield, *Primary Care: Concept, Evaluation, and Policy* (New York: Oxford University Press, 1992), 6, 213–35; B. Starfield, "Primary Care and Health: A Cross-National Comparison," *JAMA* 266, no. 16 (October 23, 1991), 2268-71; B. Starfield and L. Shi, "Policy Relevant Determinants of Health: An International Perspective," *Health Policy* 60 (2002): 201–18.

Parish Nursing in a Rural Area

Charlotte Halverson, RN, BSN,
Parish Health Ministry and Rural Health Coordinator,
Mercy Medical Center, Dubuque, Iowa

Charlotte Halverson, RN, BSN, wears two hats—that of parish health ministry and rural health coordinator for Mercy Medical Center in Dubuque, Iowa, and health training coordinator with the National Education Center for Agricultural Safety and Northeast Iowa Community College. She has been working with rural family health outreach since 1986 at Mercy Medical Center, and began the parish nurse program there the next year, with a visit from Rev. Westberg. Charlotte now works with forty parish nurses in the region, half of whom work with farm families.

Farmers work in dangerous environments, with long-term exposure to dusts and toxic chemicals, loud noise, sun and wind, and a wide variety of heavy machinery. It is an environment in which both young and old work as needed, and issues related to aging such as slower reflexes, and loss of hearing and vision can have serious consequences for safe operation of farm equipment. Farming is also a profession from which there are few vacations, and sleep deprivation is an important occupational risk factor to address, particularly at planting and harvest times. A farmer is always at his or her workplace, and the economic stressors in managing an agricultural business can be huge.

Often families live in areas where there are few medical resources available, and, while many carry health insurance, as self-employed workers their premiums are high (often costing $8000–$12,000 a year), with large copayments and deductibles. Preventative care is often not covered by their insurance.

Parish nurses working in rural churches serve as the impetus for helping the church to be community health education and resource centers. Parish nurses coordinate "miniagricultural screenings" focusing on pulmonary function and particular chronic diseases. They are available for resource referral and develop educational strategies to deal with farm-related issues, such as the high incidence of chronic lung disease and stress among farm families. Activities are aimed at all ages, includes safety day camps for kids, with puppets and age-appropriate giveaways.

Parish nurses who serve the rural families are often farm wives themselves and understand the culture well. They are able to listen as farmers share heavy burdens that others might not fully understand.

Six

Suffer the Children

Health Ministry with Babies, Young Children, and Families

Many pastors have had the sad duty of performing a funeral for a baby who has died of SIDS (Sudden Infant Death Syndrome). Happily, one of the best news items in children's health these days is fewer children are dying from SIDS, primarily because of an educational campaign with parents called "Back to Sleep," which encourages parents to place their infant child on its back to sleep on a firm mattress without blankets, comforters, quilts, pillows, or plush toys. SIDS deaths have dropped by more than 50 percent since the early 1990s, but this information still needs to reach more parents, SIDS remains the leading cause of death for children one month to one year old, according to the Nemours Foundation, which focuses on children's health.

There are a great many other health issues that can affect young children. Having an active health ministry in a congregation, with a parish nurse who helps to plan and implement health programming, is a wonderful way to help minister to families with babies and young children.

A congregational health ministry and parish nurses can play a profoundly important role in providing health information and support for healthy families. A few of these ways are listed below.

+ *Post-partum depression.* A few years ago, the country was stunned by a mother who intentionally drowned her young children. Post-partum depression, while generally less dramatic or public, can nevertheless present serious challenges for mothers and their young families. Nicki Reynolds, parish nurse at Bonhomme Presbyterian, Creve Coeur, Missouri, has worked with her congregation to develop a program called "Newborn Ministry." Its mission is to welcome the newborn into the family of faith, encourage healthy relationships within the family, and provide resources and information to the family. When a baby is born to one of the members, the parish nurse makes a visit to the hospital. Shortly after the family is home, a meal is delivered by one of the members of MOMs (Ministry of Mothers), a support group for young mothers that meets three times monthly during the school year. Around two to four weeks after the birth, a female member of the Stephen Ministry visits with a cradle cross ornament to welcome the new baby to Bonhomme Church's family. As she visits she also does an assessment of how the family is handling the new baby and all the stresses that brings. Three or four weeks after the baby comes home, the parish nurse makes a visit to deliver a folder with helpful church and resource information.

- *Immunizations.* Karen Seltzer, parish nurse at Faith Lutheran in Golden, Colorado, is co-chair of the Golden Family of Churches Health Ministries (GFCHM), which includes ten congregations in Golden: Calvary Episcopal Church, Faith Lutheran Church, First Baptist Church, First Presbyterian Church, First United Methodist Church, Golden Valley Life Church, Hillside Community Church, Mesa View Evangelical Free Church, St. Joseph's Catholic Church, and the Seventh-Day Adventist Church. The parish nurses there work with nurses in community schools to identify children who are in need of immunizations and, through local funding, are able to offer vouchers for immunizations at the local health department.

- *Safety Seats.* Motor vehicle crashes are the leading killer of children aged three to fourteen. According to the National Highway Traffic Safety Administration, child safety seats can reduce fatal injury by 71 percent for infants and by 54 percent for toddlers ages one to four. Yet seven out of ten children in child safety seats are not properly buckled in, according to *SeatCheck.org,* a national campaign to raise awareness about this issue. To make helping busy parents even easier, a number of congregations have invited their local children's hospital, police department, or fire department to offer a "child safety seat inspection" at the church. Check *www.SeatCheck.org* for a list of organizations offering this service in your area, and ask if they will come to your congregation.

• *Parenting.* Of course, many of the issues related to children's health are actually parent education issues. Parenting classes are found in many congregations, with support groups a common feature. Some parenting classes are run by counselors, others by peer groups of parents. Outside speakers can be engaged to discuss issues such as child safety.

• *Screenings.* Health fairs are a regular feature of many health ministries, and children's health issues are included in most. Screenings for height, weight, hearing, and vision are generally easy to arrange, through local health providers or through working with an organization such as Parents as Teachers. Kids, like adults, love freebies, and parish nurses are often able to arrange for donations of items such as toothbrushes, toothpaste, and other personal hygiene items. Having a special feature such as an ambulance with EMT personnel willing to "show and tell" will go a long way towards engaging children's interest in health.

• *Day-Care.* Many parish nurses provide their services to the day-care program associated with the church, training the staff on child safety and CPR, and helping with resource referral for families as needed. Parish nurse U'Essie Riley works with a day-care center affiliated with the United Church of Christ and the Presbyterian Church in East St. Louis, Illinois, called "Uni-Pres Kindercottage." She arranges for health care providers to visit the day-care center for screenings for lead levels, sickle cell anemia, hearing, vision and dental work, and to provide immunizations. She arranges for follow-up for any children who are found to need further evaluation or care.

* *Vacation Bible School* is a great time to build healthy eating and physical activity into the education program for children, and a tone can be set that is maintained through the following church school year. The Parish Nurse and Health Committee can work with the planning committee for VBS to identify snacks and games that will support the health and development of kids and work well with the theme of the week.

* *Education* is a leading factor in promoting good health and longevity, according to a study conducted by researchers at Princeton and Columbia, as reported in the *New York Times* (January 5, 2007). Many congregations provide school supplies and backpacks to families for whom the expense to purchase these would be a burden, and some have even helped to offer clothing and free haircuts.

* *Exercise* is a key element in preventing health problems for both children and adults, and a recent Harvard Medical School study found that obesity of peers (for adults) had a significant impact on obesity. While the study did not include children, the role that peers play in the development of children has been well documented. Many parish nurses are very creative in finding exercise programs for children that help to develop strong bodies and strong relationships. Beth Durban, parish nurse at St. Gabriel the Archangel Parish in St. Louis, has had outstanding success with the program "Girls on the Run," which is a national fitness program for girls aged eight to thirteen that helps them train for a 5K race. This nonprofit organization seeks to build the self-esteem, life skills, and social responsibility, and to promote social, mental, and emotional well-being. More information on "Girls on the Run" can be found at *www.girlsontherun.org*.

* *Hypertension* is on the rise, not only among adults, but also among children, due to the increase in obesity in Western countries. However, hypertension is often missed in kids,

according to a recent study reported in the *Journal of the American Medical Association* (August 22–27, 2007). Even mild to moderate high blood pressure can cause damage to the heart, kidneys, brain, and eyes over time, and puts kids at higher risk for later development of cardiovascular disease and kidney failure, among other conditions. This study found that nearly three-quarters of kids with hypertension had not been diagnosed in any of their three previous routine wellness visits. Parish nurses can help families check and log their children's blood pressure on a regular basis. Blood pressure screening: it's not only for the elderly!

Providing health information to your congregation in newsletters and bulletins is also an important role of parish nurses. Many resources exist to help them find materials online. The National Library of Medicine, in conjunction with the National Institutes of Health (NIH), has an online resource for children's health, called Medline Plus, at *www.nlm.nih.gov/medlineplus/childrenshealth .html*.

The Nemours Foundation (*www.kidshealth.org*), cited above, specializes in children's health information, and the Mayo Clinic's online health information website has an area focused on children as well: *www.mayoclinic.com/health/childrens-health/CC99999*.

The wonderful thing about working with the health of families and children is that once you get started, there is a wealth of information and resources to help you. And preventing even one loss, injury, or illness is worth all the effort in this direction of ministry to God's little ones.

Enfolded in the Arms of God

Mary Lynch, RN, Parish Nurse,
Oshawa, Ontario, Canada

One cold winter day last January, I was admitting a patient from On-cology to Rehab, and he was clutching a very colorful shawl knitted in squares by many different people. Some were loose knitters, some tight knitters, some dropped a stitch here and there, and one or two had combined colored wool in one square. All were neatly sewn together with a bright red wool. This very different patchwork-like shawl meant a lot to my new patient. He said, "All those squares were knit for me by different people praying that I would get better. It was given to me when I was dying and now I'm on my way home via Rehab to make me mobile." Three weeks later he went home with his shawl of many colors, thanking God for the knitters that gave him hope with their special prayer shawl. Later, when I visited him, he had made his shawl into a wall hanging and truly believed that in the power of prayer his life was saved.

When we first started our Prayer Shawl ministry, we received the patterns from our friends at Westminster United Church in Whitby, who were very helpful with tips. They were already making shawls for awhile and had ironed out all the knots.

Our seniors group was delighted with the challenge, wool and needles poured in, and some new knitters were helped on the way.

Shawls of all sizes came in. Father blessed them, and I had the honor of presenting them to some of our parishioners during chemotherapy. They wrapped them around their shoulders during treatments or covered their knees with the lap shawls. The people at home use them like afghans or knee wraps.

The ones I got that were like scarves were embroidered around the outside to make them bigger, and some small squares were sewn together to make a large shawl. I got one very small legal letter size, knit beautifully with very colorful, expensive wool and was at a loss for what I could do with it. The day I got it I went to visit a couple in the hospital who had twin babies. The tiny naked babies looked so cold hooked up to the IV in their incubators, and I knew then that I needed another small shawl for those special premies.

The NICU staff gave permission, the lady knitted another small shawl, and as we all prayed, the parents covered the top of the incubators with the mini prayer shawls, making them look warmer.

One shawl went to a mom who was awaiting her son's cremated remains to be returned, and another went to an oncology patient who was not sure if she was eligible for more chemotherapy. After she received her prayer shawl, her oncologist treated her and she was discharged.

One shawl went to a young immigrant girl who was devastated to discover that she was pregnant, with no family to support her. With the prayer shawl came help in finding housing, support, a baby shower, and a hand to hold as she walked the path to establish her status in Canada.

A psychiatric patient whom the staff had a hard time keeping dressed just tucked his prayer shawl around him and cried.

One of the shawls was made for a young lady in prison. I was unable to give it to her as that would be against the rules, so I gave it to her mother, who is taking care of her children.

Hostel residents really appreciate shawls, but we needed to make name tags for them. In our experience, prayer shawls without tassels are more convenient for dialysis or home chemo patients as their IV apparatus can get caught up in the extra wool.

The pleasure and hope that prayer shawls bring to our friends who have received them is heartwarming. Along with every prayer shawl goes a card explaining that as we knit, we are praying for each person that the love of God will keep them warm.

Seven

Reaching Past YouTube

Working with Teenagers

When one thinks of parish nursing, teenagers are probably not the first group that comes to mind. Teens generally are very healthy, aside from the odd cold or flu. Any chronic illnesses diagnosed in childhood, such as asthma or diabetes, are usually well managed by the teen years.

There are still many ways, however, that a congregation can be helpful to teens and their parents through health ministry. Having a parish nurse and a health cabinet to plan and implement programs is ideal. Many of the following suggestions, however, can be implemented in congregations through the leadership of others, including local resources available in the community, often for a minimal cost.

◆ *Sex education.* The teen years are "wake-up" years for sexuality, and our culture attempts to capitalize on this energy in a wide variety of ways, especially through advertising. Due to a wide variety of influences on school boards, sex education varies widely from place to place. In a world of potentially lethal sexually transmitted diseases, it is incumbent upon religious communities to share responsibility for education about sexuality with parents and schools. It is shocking to learn how often teens are unaware of the dangers of risky sexual behaviors other than intercourse. Parish nurses, who are used to dealing in a matter-of-fact manner with a wide variety of sensitive health issues, are the perfect resource persons to address these concerns with young people.

- *Healthy eating.* The World Health Organization calls child-hood and teenage obesity — which can increase the risk of illnesses such as heart disease and stroke and lead to a sig-nificantly shorter life expectancy — a global health epidemic. Approximately 15 percent of American teenagers today are overweight, with another 15 percent at risk, the highest levels in U.S. history, according to the Centers for Disease Control and Prevention (CDC). On the other hand, the media is filled with frighteningly thin people — particularly young women. Eating disorders exist among all age groups, but teens are at highest risk for developing anorexia and bulimia. Parish nurses have offered classes as part of junior high and high school church education programs on body image and eating disorders, and have helped families identify potential prob-lems and access help early. A church-wide focus on healthy eating can be a support to teens.

- *Exercise.* Recently I accompanied my daughter's Girl Scout troop on a short hike, and it was amazing to see fifth graders who could hardly walk a mile. We have convinced ourselves that it is dangerous for kids to just play around outside, and schools keep cutting back on physical education classes. Ac-cording to the CDC, 43 percent of teens watch more than two hours of TV a day. Most teens also do an hour or more of homework, and play computer and video games as well. By the time children reach their teen years, many have de-veloped habits and interests that are primarily sedentary, and teen girls are even less likely to be active than boys. Youth groups should include activities that get kids moving as often as possible.

- *Automobile accidents.* One of the most tragic tasks a pas-tor can have is ministering to grief-stricken families of car accident victims. Motor vehicle crashes, according to the Na-tional Safety Council, are the leading cause of death for young people between the ages of fifteen and twenty. A helpful pro-gram might be to have a survivor of a car accident, along with a relative of someone who died in a crash, a police officer, and an EMS technician speak to the teens. These could be separate presentations or a panel discussion, with sensitivity toward the various emotions that may be experienced by the presenters. Teens learn best by listening to peers, so the younger the presenters, the better. A teen who has survived a car accident or lost a friend would probably have the greatest impact.

- *Mental health issues.* We don't like to talk about it, but mental health issues confront a significant number of teens. Many teens are under care for ADHD and ADD, and others are diagnosed with disorders such as obsessive-compulsive disorder and bipolar disorder. Depression affects about 20 percent of teens at some time during their teenage years. Of greatest concern is the risk of suicide. The Nemours Foundation, which specializes in children's health issues, reports that the number of teen suicides continues to rise and is a leading cause of death among teenagers, particularly in the middle teen years, when hormone shifts and changing sleep patterns cause the greatest disruption. Parish nurses can arrange for screenings for risk factors for depression and other mental health issues at all-church events such as health fairs. They can also be available to help families access counselors to help with mental health issues. In some places, parish nurses have been able to help congregations arrange to have mental health care providers come to the church once a week to provide one-on-one or family counseling through a local mental health care provider.

- *Safety.* Personal safely is an issue for teens, who are given more freedom to travel around their communities on their own than are younger children. Some parish nurses have arranged for karate classes to be taught to teens, both for exercise and for personal security. They have found that the teens really enjoy the classes and show up regularly. Some have arranged for police officers to make presentations on issues such as personal safety in public spaces and date rape. A new safety issue is the rising incidence of teens playing the "choking game," in which a person obstructs the flow of oxygen to the brain (either alone or with a partner) through pressure on their carotid artery until he or she passes out, to enjoy the euphoria of oxygen returning. It has, in many hundreds if not thousands of cases a year, led to tragic death or permanent brain damage. Communication and education here are key.

* *Tobacco use.* Most lifelong smokers begin smoking in their teens, so this issue must be a priority for anyone working with the wholistic health of teens. Many parish nurses have helped people with smoking cessation programs, but few parish nurses have offered smoking prevention programs. This is a wide-open opportunity to make a difference in a community through peer support.

* *Alcohol.* The CDC found that nearly half of twelfth graders consumed alcohol in the previous month. Combined with other reckless behaviors, underage alcohol use can be deadly. It can also compound mental health issues and be a contributing factor in self-injury or other violent behavior. Teen alcohol use is almost entirely peer-related. A youth group that makes alcohol seem less attractive would certainly help. Starting a church program similar to Big Brothers or Big Sisters that pairs a young teen with an adult church member might also help to address some of the pressures that teens are under, giving them a friendly ear during these challenging years.

* *Drugs.* Drug misuse among teens can range from use of illegal drugs, such as marijuana, methamphetamine, or cocaine, to the use of medications prescribed for another person, or the use of inhalants, such as glue or other household chemicals. WebMD recommends talking with children and teens about substance abuse, and states "Involvement in church activities, YMCA programs, or youth organizations helps young people feel connected and engaged in activities and social circles that are drug- and alcohol-free." If WebMD clearly supports church activities as a drug prevention strategy, there is obviously some room for faith communities to make a positive contribution to teen health here.

* *Access to care.* It is sad to say that far too many families in the United States do not have health insurance. With changes that are currently being proposed in Congress, this may soon change significantly. In some cases, however, a family is not aware of the health insurance options available to them. Parish nurses can help ascertain whether all families in their congregation (and neighborhood) have access to health care, so that teens can receive the medical care they need. They can encourage the church to speak out for the need for health care for all. Free materials are available through nonprofit organizations such as the Robert Wood Johnson Foundation.

The bottom line is that teens face somewhat unique health issues, several of which can have profoundly serious implications. The church can play a significant role in helping these young members navigate through the special challenges these issues present.

The Positive Family Enterprise

Mary Ann Brischetto, RN, MSN,
Parish Nurse, St. Paul United Church of Christ, St. Louis

Wherever you find Mary Ann Brischetto, parish nurse at St. Paul United Church of Christ on loan as executive director of the not-for-profit Positive Family Enterprise, you will find teenagers. And little kids. And moms. For the past decade, she has served families at risk for permanently losing their children due to behaviors and situations that threaten the health and safety of the family. Not one to be easily dismissed, she has settled gang disputes and helped promote restitution due to vandalism by pulling those involved back into the community. She leads support groups for teens (as well as their mothers, as you will read below). She arranges for karate classes for teens at the church to improve their physical well-being, as well as to help reduce their fear of living in the inner city. She is also readily available to talk with teens about their concerns, often into the wee hours of the night.

Through the Positive Family Enterprise and the professionals with whom she works there, Mary Ann's program is able to provide health counseling, resource referral for needed services, and support groups for parents and for teens. She also provides food, compassionate care, and love.

Recently an advocate wrote of her work, "I am a judge in Juvenile Court. What I essentially do on a day-to-day basis is take children away from mothers who are incapable of parenting. What Mary Ann Brischetto does is nothing short of remarkable.

"Once I have removed a child from the mother, I order the mother to perform all sorts of tasks in order to get her child back. Most of the time the mother, because of either drug addiction, mental illness, homelessness, or a whole range of other factors, fails in reunification with her child. But when they work with Mary Ann, the success rate is astounding. When I refer a mother to Mary Ann, she comes into the life of the mother and transforms her. Mary Ann forces the mother to own up to her mistakes and her past and then move on in taking on the responsibilities of raising children.

"The difference in the mother from the time of her first appearance in front of me to the time when I am giving her children back to her is amazing. Mary Ann has convinced them, schooled them, and motivated mothers to become, quite simply, just better persons. The philosophy of unconditional love partnered with strict discipline works miracles."

Parish nurses, clergy, and other health ministers share unconditional love and witness miracles every day!

Eight

Aging in Community

Supporting Care of the Elderly

If it seems like you have been making a lot of hospital calls lately, you probably have been. If it seems like you have been talking with a lot of older people with health concerns lately, the same growing trend holds true.

Americans are living longer than ever before, and the numbers of seniors are growing. More of us are living with one, and often more, chronic illnesses. Families are less likely to all live in one area than they were in past generations, and people are looking to the churches for help.

Parish nurses and other health ministers can play a role in helping churches to address the considerable needs for care, both of the elderly who have health concerns, and of their caregivers.

Consider these facts:

We are living longer, and more of us are older. According to the National Center for Health Statistics, the life expectancy for a child born today is nearly seventy-eight years. A study at the RAND Center found that by 2030, one-fifth of the U.S. population will be over the age of sixty-five.

We are, however, often living with chronic illness. As mentioned in chapter 5 on working with adults, 45 percent of the U.S. population has a chronic medical condition, and about half of those (60 million people) have more than one chronic condition. Eighty-three percent of individuals over age sixty-five have multiple chronic conditions and nearly one-quarter of that group (23 percent) has five or more chronic conditions.

So when you think that *more than three-quarters of the seniors in your congregation have more than one chronic health condition,* and many of them are women living alone who may have limited financial resources, it is easy to see that they, their families, and you need support. One way to help coordinate outreach to these seniors and their families is through the health ministry of parish nursing.

Here are ten ways a parish nurse can help a congregation care for its elderly members who have health issues:

1. *Help with understanding current health status.* Parish nurses can accompany elderly parishioners on a doctor's visit in order to help interpret what is said. This is generally of value both for the patient, who has an extra set of ears, and for the doctor, who has someone there who can reinforce what is being shared. As long as the individual gives permission for the nurse to be there (we suggest a written form, which the parish nurse would keep on file), the doctor will almost always allow this. With this permission, there is no violation of privacy of personal health information.

2. *Help with understanding current medications.* A parish nurse can look at an elderly person's prescribed medications (and drugs that are in their medicine cabinet) to see if an outside appraisal by a pharmacist or physician might be needed in order to avoid drug interactions.

3. *Help staying compliant with treatment.* A parish nurse can follow up with seniors to be sure that they are taking their prescribed medications as directed, and getting to any therapy or treatments they might need.

4. *Help with accessing needed services.* Close to half (46 percent) of all patients in America do not receive the recommended course of care for their treatment, according to a study published in the *New England Journal of Medicine* (vol. 354, no. 11 [2006]: 1147–56.) A parish nurse can help patients ask questions about their treatment or about another opinion.

5. *Help with finding needed support.* A parish nurse can evaluate programs in the community that provide services to seniors with health needs and help those individuals and their families choose the programs that best fit their needs and budgets.

6. *Help with understanding health insurance coverage.* It is often difficult enough to decipher the explanation of benefits that someone without major health concerns receives. When it is complicated by multiple conditions, multiple providers, and sometimes multiple insurers beyond Medicare, it is helpful to have an advocate, such as a parish nurse, to help navigate through the morass of paperwork. By helping people better understand their options, parish nurses can help reduce the fear that often accompanies the cost of health services.

7. *Help with understanding advance directives.* Patients may fear that they will receive unwanted treatment should they become incapacitated. A parish nurse can provide information to the congregation or to individuals on advanced directives or living wills, or can arrange for another professional to provide that information free of charge.

8. *Help with staying active.* A parish nurse can oversee exercise programs for people with health conditions, such as "armchair" exercise programs, or supervised walking programs at the church for people who would not feel safe walking alone.

9. *Help with staying connected.* A parish nurse can help provide socialization for elders who may be at risk for becoming homebound without the health support that a health ministry can provide. For example, a person who has recovered from a broken hip may be reluctant to leave home alone, but may be more willing to start getting out again with the assistance of a nurse for a program at church to meet with friends.

10. *Help with financial constraints.* An important factor in patient health is the prohibitive cost of medications or needed

therapies, not all of which are covered by Medicare or Medicaid. Parish nurses can help parishioners (who may be too embarrassed to ask for help) access programs that provide medications, medical appliances, or needed medical services at reduced rates.

Aging is hard enough. Aging alone, without the support of a caring community equipped to provide sensitive, helpful support, is a fate worse than death. The church has always cared for the elderly. Intentional health ministry helps even more.

A Moment of Sharing Life

Tamara Zujewskyj, RN, BScN, MScN,
Parish Nurse, Edmonton Moravian Church,
Edmonton, Alberta, Canada

Our meeting...her wide blue eyes softly gaze at a space between here and somewhere else. The tilt of her head and her sloping shoulders define a resignation to what surrounds her. Her hands folded together pray a lonely prayer. Her silvery white locks hint of an undaunted spirit. She sits alone at her table, from which three of her companions have long departed, as if waiting for something to happen, for her turn at something she doesn't remember.

I enter her space, honoring her presence. My heart wells up into my throat, and a wave of emotion washes over me. I don't want to startle her and want so much to connect my eyes with hers to feel her presence within me. As I draw nearer she continues to stay in her space. Only my light touch on her arm brings her closer. Her eyes meet mine and a smile touches the corner of her mouth. I speak her name. She searches for recognition. Her words say to me: "I have not seen you for a long time," and I notice words falling from my mouth: "Yes, I am Tamara, the nurse from the Moravian Church." I want to ease the way for her memory, and she repeats "Moravian Church" with a sigh that comes from somewhere deep inside her. I feel the warm breath from her mouth as she speaks the words. It is as if somewhere from inside her, her spirit has stirred and I touched a place that remembers.

"May I stay with you awhile?" I say to her wide blue eyes. "Yes," she answers from somewhere between...between where I sit and where she has been.

We spend some time looking at the pictures scattered around the room. Sometimes she stops at one and searches for the words that would express her thought or feeling, but the words won't listen and insist on mixing her up. She sighs as if this deeper breath would bring her closer to what she wants to say. We smile at each other and a warmth spreads throughout my body. The smile touches each of us and I wonder what she feels beneath hers. I touch her hand, and she grasps mine initially as if she is grasping something she doesn't want to let go.

I ask her if she would like to pray, and her eyes slip into that space where she was on my arrival. "Would you like to say the Lord's Prayer with me?" Her eyes, full of recognition, touch mine as she says, "You say it." As I say the words in prayer, her mouth moves, and it seems for me for a moment that the words are actually coming from her.

We have been together for a moment in eternity. In the eternity of God's time where all words we need are always there. I say my farewells and move closer with her permission to give her a hug and kiss. Her body falls into mine as if with relief and she plants a kiss on my cheek as I plant one on hers. For a moment there is calm and comfort and she whispers, "That feels so good." I say to her, "Indeed it does."

And so once again, she has affirmed for me that there is awe and wonder in the communion of fellow travelers of God's world.

Nine

Thirty-Five Years of Care
Caring for the Caregiver

Many adults who have chronic health conditions are being cared for by a spouse who may have health concerns of his or her own. When a spouse dies or when the senior has been unmarried or is divorced, much of that care falls to a family member, usually a daughter or niece, who many times is caring for her own children at the same time. That person may live nearby or many miles away.

Judith Steinberg Turiel, a health writer who found herself caring for her aging mother who suffered from dementia, learned that the average American woman can expect to spend eighteen years helping aging parents and other relatives, along with seventeen years caring for her own children. Eighty percent of the 9 million Americans living alone are women who have spent their lives caring for family, regardless of whether they have also worked outside the home.[1]

Here are some ways that parish nurses can help with care for the caregivers.

- Parish nurses can help explain the health condition of the loved one. They have fewer time constraints than most health professionals who are working within health systems.

- Parish nurses can help recruit and train lay volunteers in the congregation to help provide simple needed services — such as transportation, meals, or light housekeeping.

- Parish nurses can be available for consultation about services, such as adult day care, home health care, or nursing homes.

- Parish nurses can help identify good sources of respite care, so that caregivers can have some time for relaxation or to run needed errands. Parish nurses may know of funding sources to pay for respite care.

- Sometimes the only person a caregiver can leave a loved one with is a nurse — and parish nurses sometimes provide respite care for caregivers.

- Parish nurses can develop caregiver support groups that can provide needed breaks and socialization for the caregivers.

- Some parish nurses have worked closely with the Faith in Action Program of the Robert Wood Johnson Foundation to develop a volunteer interfaith caregivers program, which provides support to families where a member has a chronic, debilitating illness.

- Parish nurses can be a listening ear for the caregiver and are available at times when other health professionals do not have office hours. Having a nurse to talk to can be a great relief.

- Parish nurses can screen the caregiver on a regular basis for hypertension and arrange for other care as needed.

- Parish nurses can help a caregiver reintegrate back into the church after her or his loved one dies. Caregivers often want to start back to church by volunteering to help with the congregation's health ministry. They are eager to "give back" some of what they received.

There are myriad ways for parish nurses and other health ministers to be helpful to the life of a congregation and its many members, including the elderly with health concerns and their caregivers. Given the trends with aging and illness, all help is greatly needed.

Notes

1. Judith Steinberg Turiel, *Our Parents, Ourselves: How American Health Care Imperils Middle Age and Beyond* (Berkeley: University of California Press, 2005), 45.

Separated by Miles, Joined by Care

Ellen Van Arsdale, Congregational Nurse,
Desert Palms Presbyterian Church, Sun City West, Arizona

Bud is an eighty-eight-year-old gentleman, living in Sun City West, Arizona. He has been widowed since 1993, but maintains an active lifestyle despite living alone. He enjoys golf and stamp collecting and has traveled extensively. He attends worship on a regular basis. He has two loving children, both of whom live out of state. He has enjoyed good health, with the only major illness being scarlet fever at age eighteen.

In May of 2006, Bud was hospitalized for what he thought would be a minor surgical procedure to insert a pacemaker. He was told that he suffered cardiac arrhythmia which was causing some fatigue. Approximately one week following the procedure he returned home but did not feel like himself. He shared his concerns with his daughter, Nancy, who called the congregational nurse, Ellen. In Bud's words, he felt alone, frightened, helpless, and perplexed as to why he still felt so awful. He went to the ER with Ellen and after numerous tests was sent home. It soon became apparent to Bud, Ellen, and Nancy that further evaluation was needed. Bud was hospitalized and then sent to an assisted living unit. When he was ready to return home, additional in-home help was found. He is now feeling like himself and returning to the activities he enjoys.

"I didn't really feel depressed," said Bud, "but I simply could not put my finger on what was wrong. I was so appreciative of the support from my congregation and the congregational nurse. She was someone I could count on. I knew that the church cared about my welfare. Ellen and Nancy worked as a team in communicating what was happening. Nancy's frequent visits were so important to me, but when she could not be here, I knew that Ellen was here. I no longer feel helpless or hopeless and look forward to time spent with family and friends. I am glad that our church has a congregational nurse."

Ellen has this to share about her experience. "Bud was one of the most outgoing eighty-eight-year-olds I have met in my work with older adults. I first met him while making hospital rounds and found him to be a man of varied interests and talents. I was surprised to get the call from Nancy asking me to see him in his home and subsequently to make a trip to the ER. Clearly, all was not well. I hesitated to leave Bud alone but told him I would check on him daily. Fortunately for Bud, Nancy was able to travel to his home, and it soon became clear to her as well that further evaluation was needed. I continued to make frequent visits to the hospital and then to the assisted living unit. Nancy and I were in nearly daily communication, and she left no stone unturned in seeking resources for her father. I suggested she inquire about a teleconference call, which would allow her and her brother to listen in on a case conference and ask questions as well. This worked well and saved them an additional trip. I could not have asked for a more cooperative family to work with and was thrilled with the outcome. I will continue to keep in touch with Bud but feel that he has had a very positive outcome to what could have been a debilitating physical condition."

Nancy writes: "I know my dad feels enormously grateful for Ellen's help and attention, but I feel that *I* benefited the most! It's difficult to be fifteen hundred miles away when your sole surviving parent is ailing. I don't recall how Ellen's name came to me, but I telephoned her after my father returned home from surgery. She visited him and was my salvation a few days later when he began having chest pains. One phone call from me, and Ellen picked him up and drove him to the hospital, waiting with him in the ER while tests were run and evaluated — a five-hour ordeal! Ellen was the 'health care professional' member of our small, family-based 'team' with whom I communicated by email during my dad's tribulations. His heretofore unknown 'parish nurse' lent her considerable strength and attention to us during what turned out to be a three-month road to recovery. Ellen visited my father often. . . . She genially but perceptively listened to his complaints, queried his doctors, and shared her observations about him with me on the phone and by email. She answered millions of little questions doctors don't have time for, but whose answers make a lot of difference to patients. She was invaluable in sharing resources as I built a list of caregivers and services and advised me well on navigating the insurance system. She reminded me of Bud's important 'patient rights' and found creative ways to keep everyone in the loop. The comfort I felt knowing Ellen was there if my dad needed her was enormous. Her medical background was reassuring to me, especially tempered with the church values we share; I know she truly cares about my father, as a fellow congregant needing her skills, and now, as a friend. That combination is the great and special gift a parish nurse has to offer her or his church: a commitment to good health made possible by years of professional nursing experience, suffused with Christian values of love and service. Ellen's sensitive ministrations helped my father recover with his dignity intact. Thank you, dear Ellen."

Ten

When Did We See You?

Caring for the Dying

One out of every eight people in America today is over sixty-five and by 2030, that ratio will be one in five (World Bank, 2005). The American Nurses Association estimates there are 2.5 million nurses in the United States, but according to a 2004 report by the U.S. Bureau of Labor Statistics, 1 million new and replacement nurses will be needed by 2012. Given the growing numbers of the aging and the declining supply of health care professionals (doctors will be in short supply as well), who will care for the dying?

Today, nurses are leaving hospitals for reasons such as stress, injury, and burnout, yet many of those same nurses are looking to the church as a place to care for neighbors in a wholistic way, as Jesus commanded:

> "Lord, when was it that we saw you hungry and gave you food, or thirsty and gave you something to drink? And when was it that we saw you a stranger and welcomed you, or naked and gave you clothing? And when was it that we saw you sick or in prison and visited you?" And the king will answer them, "Truly, I tell you, just as you did it to one of the least of these who are members of my family, you did it to me." (Matthew 25:37b–40)

These nurses, as part of the ministry team, can be of great help to terminally ill parishioners and their families. Few times of life are as fearsome as the dying journey. Here are some of the ways parish nurses can assist with a church's health ministry.

Health Education

♦ *Health information.* Parish nurses can provide education to individuals and groups about specific health conditions, such as diabetes, heart disease, cancer, and other potentially life-threatening conditions. In most health care settings today, patients have little time with their doctor, and care between specialists is often fragmented. Parish nurses have the flexibility and opportunity to spend more time with parishioners in a variety of settings — at church, in the hospital, in a nursing home, or at home.

♦ *Hospice.* Parish nurses can provide congregants with information about hospice, so that patients can discuss this option early on with their physicians and indicate they might have an interest in using the services of hospice should their condition so warrant. Only one-quarter of Americans who died in 2002 used the services of hospice,[1] but many others could likely have done so had they been aware of their options earlier.

♦ *Death and dying.* Most parish nurses have been staff nurses for several years before becoming a parish nurse and are familiar with the physical processes of dying. They can help parishioners and their families understand the changes that a body goes through as death approaches, and can provide reassurance and support. They can advocate pain management, as pain is often one of the most feared aspects of dying.

♦ *Advanced directives.* Parish nurses can encourage all parishioners to have a "Living Will," or "Advanced Directives," which explain the wishes of a patient for health care should he or she be unable to communicate directly. With the parishioner's permission, the parish nurse can keep a copy of these in her file, for use if necessary.

♦ *Advanced planning.* Some parish nurses have facilitated classes on end-of-life issues that begin with clergy discussing death and dying from a theological point of view and move toward logistical matters, such as how to make arrangements with a funeral home, so that a family is not taken by surprise and understands each loved one's wishes.

+ *Organ donation.* While every effort is made to save the life of someone who is ill, parish nurses can provide information to congregations about how donation of organs after death can positively affect the lives of others. (See p. 122 for more information.)

Health Counseling

+ *Health status.* "Knowledge is power," the saying goes, and sometimes having a better understanding of one's health status helps one to feel more comfortable with a diagnosis and prognosis. Parish nurses have time to discuss health issues with individual parishioners in a variety of settings.

+ *Health options.* Sometimes having someone with whom to discuss and weigh options is important. While parish nurses do not provide medical diagnoses or prescribe treatments, they are generally willing to accompany parishioners to the doctor, encourage them to ask questions, and help them understand and access their health care options.

+ *Nutrition.* Generally, a person who is dying has little interest in food. A parish nurse can help parishioners and their families understand what might be helpful when considering nutrition at the end of life.

+ *Other services.* Parish nurses can help a family evaluate services for those nearing the end of life, such as nursing homes, hospice programs, respite care, and other home-based services.

+ *Support groups.* Parish nurses can help to develop support groups for individuals with life-threatening illnesses, such as cancer or Parkinson's disease. They can also help to facilitate support groups for caregivers, as well as for grief support.

Coordination of Volunteers

♦ *Visitation.* A parish nurse ministry is not a ministry of an individual, but rather a part of the entire church's health ministry.
Participation by others, therefore, is central to the vitality of
this work. Parish nurses can prepare volunteers to visit the
sick and dying and to help support the family. No one should
have to die alone.

♦ *Meals.* Volunteers can help to provide light meals for the
family.

♦ *Housekeeping.* Light housekeeping may be a support to the
person who is dying, or his or her family, and volunteers can
help in this regard.

♦ *Errands.* Volunteers are often able to run brief errands for
others, such as going to the grocery store.

Integration of Faith and Health

Those involved in health ministry often encourage the dying
and their families to find places of comfort and hope in ways
that have been meaningful to them over the years, for example,
through being in a garden (or near a window that looks out
over a garden), listening to music, or reading favorite poetry. Of
course, parish nurses, like clergy, encourage and support prayer
and meditation.

No member of a faith community who is facing death should
face dying in fear and loneliness. Each member of the Body of
Christ is precious and made in the image of God. Parish nursing
is one vital way for the church to respond to the question, "When
did we see you . . . ?"

Notes

1. Beth Han et al., "Trends: National Trends in Adult Hospice Use:
1991–1992 to 1999–2000," *Health Affairs* 25, no. 3 (May–June 2006):
792–99.

My Parish Nurse

Christine Cosnowski, RN, MSA,
Faith Community Nurse, Member of the Detroit
Parish Nurse Network of Southeast Michigan
by Helene King

My parish nurse is indispensable! She is indispensable to the community, the church, and the individual.

For the community, my parish nurse helps arrange blood drives, teaches CPR, helps churches procure AEDs (automatic external defibrillators), drives the elderly to doctor's appointments and beyond. She also belongs to many organizations that enable her to bring many different people together to meet their individual and unique needs. Such needs might be grief counseling or, in my case, finding a recipient for our no-longer-needed wheelchair ramp.

For the church, my parish nurse has monthly blood pressure clinics, arranges for flu shots, writes a timely and very informative article for the newsletter, teaches CPR and babysitting classes, teaches the youth about health issues, makes presentations to the Stephen Ministry training, and much more.

For the individual, my parish nurse makes home visits to the ill, the recovering, and the shut-ins. She also makes hospital visits and many, many follow-up phone calls. My parish nurse provides support for mind, body, and spirit, finds medical equipment for loan, helps decipher medical and pharmaceutical terms and issues, and answers questions. Where does she find the time?

And then there are those special individual moments. I certainly have shared many with my parish nurse. I would like to share one with you. When my parish nurse came to our church, it was two months before my husband, Terry, died from kidney cancer. I had been introduced to her but did not avail myself of her services. She was new, and I tend to do things on my own.

Then came the night when Terry was taken to Henry Ford Hospital, Downtown Detroit. I was there alone. The staff approached me and offered hospice care for him. Extenuating circumstances made it a very difficult decision. At that moment, I looked up and saw a familiar face. I didn't immediately identify her, but recognized the face. As she approached, I realized it was my parish nurse. At 9:00 p.m., she had driven to Downtown Detroit to be with me — with me — so that I would not be alone in making that decision. Her support and comfort were a much appreciated blessing. She was indeed an angel sent by God to walk that path with me.

Eleven

A Spirit of Shalom
Addressing Mental Health Needs

Health and wholeness, we claim in faith communities, is not simply the absence of disease. It more, much more, perhaps encompassed best as a spirit of *shalom*. As I am sure you know, *shalom* is a traditional Hebrew greeting meaning both "welcome" and "goodbye" (God be with you) as well as "peace" and "well-being."

It is hard, however, to have a spirit of well-being when dealing with a mental health concern, despite good physical health. "Isolation is not just a matter of kilometers," says Sarah James, a young woman from Australia who suffers from mental illness as she seeks to educate others about the plight of teens with similar issues.

Statistics show that mental health issues are relatively common among all age groups:[1]

- More than 28 percent of Americans have a mental disorder in any given one-year period.

- About 3 percent of the adult population experiences severe mental disorders in any one-year period.

- About 2 percent of adults have a serious mental illness.

- More than 3 million people have mental retardation. About one-third of those individuals live in institutional settings.

- The lifetime prevalence of post-traumatic stress disorder for adults is 6.8 percent, with women twice as likely to experience PTSD (at 10.5 percent) than men (5 percent) due to a higher incidence of domestic violence and sexual trauma.

- Between 3 percent and 5 percent of children have ADHD, approximately 2 million children in the United States.

- Approximately 1 in 150 children have an Autism Spectrum Disorder.

- Depression affects approximately 5 percent of all adults at some time in their lives, and approximately 40 percent of those individuals will experience clinical depression.

- Dementia or a disease such as Alzheimer's can have profound impact on the life of elderly people and their families, and these conditions are often incorrectly diagnosed or treated.

That means that in a Sunday School of twenty-five to thirty children, it is likely that at least one child will have Attention Deficit Hyperactivity Disorder. Another youth may have autism. One in a dozen women or and a few men may be experiencing mental health issues related to an earlier trauma. Several people in your congregation may be experiencing depression at any given time. Others may be caring for people living with dementia or Alzheimer's. Mental health issues need to be discussed and planned for in a health ministry of a congregation.

Some of the mental health issues experienced by parishioners can be easily treated and managed. Other disorders experienced by millions of Americans are far more serious and long-lasting. Unfortunately, the stigma attached to mental health issues is greater than that attached to most physical ailments, with the possible exception of sexually transmitted diseases or other health concerns related to sexuality. Organizations such as the National Alliance on Mental Illness sponsors faith-based initiatives to help congregations educate themselves on how to help individuals and families facing mental health concerns.

Alcohol and drug addiction are physical *and* mental health concerns. Organizations such as Committed Caring Faith Communities in St. Louis have brought together clergy, parish nurses, and other faith community members to bring these issues to the forefront of awareness in congregational settings. Sharon Ema, RN, parish nurse and minister of health and wellness at

Concordia Lutheran Church in Kirkwood, Missouri, has been particularly active in educating her congregation and community about this issue through this organization.

Developmental disabilities, too, call faith communities to move beyond simply physical and spiritual well-being. People living with developmental disabilities present different opportunities for inclusion. The First United Methodist Church in Vermillion, South Dakota, is a congregation where several residents of a group home for adults with mental retardation and/or developmental disabilities attend worship regularly. On a recent visit there, I observed Rev. Brook McBride, the minister in that congregation, welcoming their spoken prayers, including requests to have "Happy Birthday" sung in honor of their own birthdays. Rev. McBride comfortably acknowledged their presence and promised to honor their request later in the service, which he did. The congregation, through his leadership, was prepared for difference and was able to include those whose needs for community were different from the norm.

Evangelical United Church of Christ in Webster Groves, Missouri, often welcomes a choir composed of adults with developmental disabilities from the nearby Emmaus Homes to sing and stay for lunch following the service. The pastor, Rev. Katherine Hawker, is a board member at Emmaus, encouraging their regular participation with the congregation.

Here are a few observations from congregations that have been successful in outreach and care to people with mental health concerns:

Variety is the spice of life, but regularity is an anchor for many with mental health issues. Many mental health conditions are severely disorienting and make day-to-day living more challenging. For a person living with autism or post-traumatic stress disorder, for example, having certain elements in the worship service that are always the same is a great comfort. (It probably is to most of the rest of us, as well.)

Visual elements in worship encourage participation for those who have trouble with reading the bulletin. Having a screen with different visual elements available is a support to people who may have difficulty with language, such as some children with autism, Down syndrome, or other special needs.

Families who have loved ones with challenging conditions such as dementia or severe autism may be particularly stressed. They may need pastoral care — often! Some congregations have started support groups for caregivers of people with dementia or other mental health concerns. Access to different support groups can be open to congregations and neighbors throughout the community. There is no need to reinvent the wheel. The wonderful thing about health ministers is that they network.

Don't expect families who have a loved one living with a mental health concern to join regular committees. You can invite them to participate, but also offer episodic opportunities to volunteer. They may be very, very tired.

How can parish nurses help?

Resources. Parish nurses can help find needed resources for people living with mental health concerns. Unless your family has experienced autism, PTSD, or Alzheimer's with a family member, you probably don't realize the extent that those conditions can tax an individual and a family system. One parish nurse helped a young man with obsessive-compulsive disorder, who would not leave his parents' house because of his need to wash his hands. She found him a mental health provider and arranged transportation for him so that he did not need to touch anything in order to get there. He has made amazing progress and is now socializing and working toward getting employment.

Education. Parish nurses can put articles on mental health issues in the church bulletin or newsletter. They also can arrange for mental health professionals to speak on various topics, helping people feel that it is okay to discuss mental health and to seek help in finding appropriate support and services.

Screening. Parish nurses also can provide rudimentary screening for certain mental health related issues, such as depression, as part of a health fair. They can also help people access needed services for screenings through mental health providers.

Help with Caregiving. Parish nurses can visit families where caregiving is needed and help arrange for needed services, such as meals, visiting, or transportation, through coordination of volunteers. Parish nurses can help arrange for respite care for caregivers of people whose family members must be supervised because of their mental health concern.

Spiritual Care. Parish nurses can help identify parishioners in need of spiritual care. They can then pass on requests for spiritual care to the pastor and will also pray with parishioners who are seeking God in their distress.

Mental health issues are not a matter of simple willpower or "time healing all wounds." A community of care is one that is willing, like Jesus, to walk with those who are troubled in spirit, bringing them a "spirit of shalom."

Notes

1. Statistics from the National Institute of Mental Health, the National Institute on Disability and Rehabilitation Research, the National Dissemination Center for Children with Disabilities, the American Association on Health and Disability, the Centers for Disease Control and Prevention, the United States Department of Veterans Affairs, and the American Psychiatric Association.

HEALTH MINISTRY IN ACTION

Parish Nursing Outcome: Lives Intertwined

Carol Lemon, RN, Member of the Parish Nurse Coalition of the Greater Lehigh Valley, and Initiative of Sacred Heart Hospital in Allentown, Pennsylvania
by Mary O'Donnell-Miller, Health Minister,
St. Nicholas Roman Catholic Church,
Berlinsville, Pennsylvania

Lorraine, a fifty-one-year-old female with Down syndrome, is delightful, loving, and engaging. When her parents became unable to care for her any longer, the state guided her family to place Lorraine in a group home where sedating medications were used to manage her behaviors. In her three years there Lorraine became lethargic and less interactive; she was unable to hold her head up, sleeping more and drooling at the mouth. She became inactive and gained weight. Her brother, not consulted about the changes in her medications, became concerned. Ron, a deeply caring and spiritual man, believes strongly in the values instilled in him by his mother: family should take care of family. He decided to take Lorraine home to live with him.

Ron's parish nurse, Carol Lemon, at Blessed Virgin Mary of Colesville, assisted Ron and Lorraine in the transition. First, a comprehensive physical evaluation was completed by the Eastern Pennsylvania Down Syndrome Center. Carol attended the interview as an advocate. She utilized her parish connections with Share-Care Faith in Action for volunteers to provide friendship and respite. She spoke with the Diocese of Allentown about admission to Mercy Special Learning Center for the over twenty-one group; Lorraine is on the waiting list. Ron helped find state funding to hire caregivers when he needs to be away and arranged for Lorraine to start exercise classes. She has lost twenty pounds. Carol visits, takes her for walks, and accompanies her to well-woman appointments. But more than these concrete things, Carol provides a nurturing relationship that brings healing. Through spiritual and emotional support, she empowers and enables Lorraine and Ron to make wholistic health care decisions.

Carol strongly believes in parish nursing's role in health and healing. She promotes early intervention and wellness. One of her guiding principles for the practice of parish nursing comes from the late Father Finnegan, one of the founding fathers of parish nursing in the Lehigh Valley: the principle of hospitality is the beginning of community. She takes that with her on all her visits, believing in relationship health as a focal point for physical, psychological, and spiritual health.

When I asked Lorraine what Carol does that helps her, her face lit up and she resolutely said, "She takes me out to lunch," as she patted her belly. Lorraine is now an active member in the church community as a greeter at Mass with the ministers of hospitality at the door, in passing the collection basket, and in bringing gifts to the altar. She enjoys life, spending time with friends, doing puzzles, going to the gym, and going out to lunch. She is thriving and is once again a delightful, loving, and engaging person.

Twelve

As You Have Done to the Least of These, You Have Done to Me
Health Advocacy

In May 2003, the Congressional Budget Office released a report stating that nearly 60 million non-elderly American children and adults did not have health insurance coverage during at least part of the year.[1] This is nearly one quarter of all children and working-age adults in this country! Of course, many of those people are parishioners in various congregations, or members of other faith groups in the United States. What can an individual congregation do to address this discrepancy in access to care that exists among its membership and neighbors? What can an individual congregation do to address other health issues that cry out for advocacy?

Jesus said, "As you did it to one of the least of these my brethren, you did it to me" (Matt. 25:40b). Caring for those falling through the cracks is an important part of the church's mandate to preach, teach, *and* heal. Working in partnership with a parish nurse, who serves as a member of the staff and has a primary role as health advocate, congregations can help to address access to care and other issues related to health and social justice.

The Role of Advocate

A parish nurse's specific assignments within the ministry of a congregation are usually decided in consultation with other church leaders and/or a "health cabinet" in the parish. Together, they may design an outreach ministry to the surrounding neighborhood or a very specialized ministry, such as within a school. Most parishes, however, prefer that the parish nurse serve broadly in response to the varied needs of the congregation and neighborhood, and advocacy is a very important piece of that response.

When considering advocacy in parish nursing, one must also define what is meant by health. "Health," in the context of parish nursing, is broadly interpreted to mean healthy and healing relationships with God, family, faith communities, society, and creation, forged by fostering physical, emotional, spiritual, and social harmony. In other words, you aren't healthy if you don't have enough food to eat, adequate housing, and safe streets to walk down. Health is more than just the absence of disease or living fully within the limitations of a chronic or terminal disease. It is a wholistic approach to life and relationships.

Listed below are several ways in which the parish nurse can make an important contribution as an advocate.

1. *Helping to obtain access to care.* As mentioned above, nearly 60 million American children and working-age adults do not have health insurance at some point during the year. Parish nurses can help identify health insurance programs for which families might be eligible. For example, in Missouri currently, children living in families who earn up to 300 percent of the federal poverty level are eligible for health insurance coverage. Parish nurses can help educate parishioners about their options, and if coverage is simply not available or affordable, they can often help parishioners obtain services for a reduced fee or at no cost. Rev. Susan Naylor, a parish nurse and deacon at Emmanuel Lutheran Church in Webster Groves, spent several years as a parish nurse advocate for Bosnian refugees in downtown St. Louis, helping people access providers who would accept Medicaid managed care.

2. *Serving as a health navigator.* Even for parishioners with good health insurance, finding one's way through the morass

of physicians, clinics, hospitals, and paperwork (including the new Medicare D provisions) can be daunting, especially for the elderly. In addition, patients may not necessarily be aware of all their options. A parish nurse helps parishioners understand what questions to ask to be fully informed about their options for services and treatment.

3. *Serving as a patient advocate in the health care system.* The Rev. Dr. Richard Ellerbrake, president emeritus of Deaconess Health System in St. Louis, would tell us that our nation's "health care system" is neither — it focuses on illness care, and the "system" is either unfinished or broken. To illustrate this point at the Westberg Symposium in 2002, Rev. Dr. Ellerbrake quoted Dr. William Jarvis of the Centers for Disease Control and Prevention, who announced that nearly 2 million patients annually get an infection while being treated in the hospital for another illness or injury. The CDC says that in the year 2000, ninety thousand of those patients died. These "nosocomial" infections are this nation's fourth most common cause of death, and account for more fatalities than car accidents and homicides combined.

There have also been a number of stories about residents who have been neglected or harmed while in the care of a nursing home. A parish nurse can act as an advocate for patients in hospitals and nursing homes, to help monitor their care and to encourage the patient and their family to speak up when they are concerned about some aspect of treatment.

4. *Working to acquire needed services in a community.* What if there are no providers of a needed service in a community? For example, in the St. Louis metropolitan area, there are very few dentists willing to provide care to children on Medicaid. Parish nurses have mobilized to address these concerns in a number of ways: one arranged for the local health department to come to the afterschool program with which she worked, where they provided sealants to children at no cost. Another parish nurse, Betty Leppard, who serves at

St. Paul United Church of Christ in Belleville, arranged for
children in her neighborhood to be bussed to a dentist's office
in the next town. And a number of parish nurses are connect-
ing with a program called "Smiles Across America," which
connects children and providers. Has the problem been elim-
inated? Not yet! But parish nurses are raising awareness
about the issue and improving the dental health of many
children.

5. *Mobilizing for the health of neighbors.* Parish nurses can
work together with parishioners to reach out into the community to improve the health of their neighbors. The Positive
Family Enterprise at St. Paul's United Church of Christ in
St. Louis is led by Mary Ann Brischetto. Mary Ann facilitates classes on parenting and life management skills for
families who are falling through the cracks. Many of the
families in the program have been referred through St. Louis
City Family Court, with positive outcomes and rave reviews
from both the participants and the court. This program is
helping families learn the skills they need to care for their
children and find stable housing, employment, and health
care. One of the program's graduates, Bess, is a mother of
three kids aged eight through sixteen, and through the Positive Family Enterprise she found safe housing and a job as
a paraprofessional that she has kept for over eight years (a
job that provides health benefits for her family, as well). Her
kids are all in school and looking forward to healthy fu-
tures of their own. (See the story on p. 73 for more on this
outreach.)

6. *Raising awareness of legislative issues related to health.*
While parish nurses certainly cannot tell parishioners what
to think or how to vote, they can educate parishioners
about health-related issues being addressed by lawmakers
and can encourage action. Time and time again we have
been told that even a few letters or calls to legislators make
a difference. Parish nurses have helped educate parishioners
about proposed legislation related to changes in Medicaid

coverage, the use and carrying of weapons, health insurance coverage for children, and use of seatbelts, among other issues.

7. *Advocating for environmental health concerns.* Several of the parish nurses in St. Louis work in neighborhoods where nearly 40 percent of the children test positive for lead poisoning. Some of the other areas in which parish nurses work have environmental toxins in the ground, water, or air. Global warming may become an environmental threat to us all. Parish nurses help educate parishioners and neighbors about environmental health concerns and help them know what choices they have with which to respond. For example, parish nurses working in areas where there are high levels of exposure to lead paint will help families get their children tested for lead poisoning, help them obtain treatment if necessary, help them identify sources to perform lead abatement, and help them find alternative housing if necessary. A number of parish nurses are also in contact with their legislators about these issues and encourage others to speak with theirs as well.

8. *Working for others in developing countries.* Those who are drawn to parish nursing often find it absorbs their entire lives, and they end up traveling on mission trips to help with the health-related concerns in developing countries as well. They often talk pastors and other parishioners into going with them, working on such projects as building schools and bridges, supplying water purifiers, and helping with projects that will develop the local economies to improve the health of the entire community. To arrange such travel parish nurses generally work through an organized group, such as CEPAD (a ministry of the Protestant churches of Nicaragua working together in emergency relief, peacemaking, and development), or a denominationally related mission organization. Upon their return, they and the other participants on such trips become advocates for the people with whom they worked. (See chapter 4 for another example of international

health ministry outreach through parish nurse and clergy partnerships.)

Parish nursing, only two decades old, is growing rapidly. Today the ministry of a parish nurse includes far more than blood pressure screenings and telling people to exercise and eat more fruits and vegetables. For a congregation interested in expanding its ministries to the "least of these," parish nursing is an effective model for change.

Notes

1. "How Many People Lack Health Insurance and For How Long?" Economic and Budget Issue Brief, Congressional Budget Office, May 12, 2003. The number of uninsured at any given time during a year has risen to nearly 16 percent of the population, according to the study by DeNavas-Walt, C. B. Proctor, and C. H. Lee, *Income, Poverty, and Health Insurance Coverage in the United States: 2005* (Washington, DC: U.S. Census Bureau, August 2006).

A Year in the Life of a New Parish Nurse

Peg D'Ambrosio, Parish Nurse,
St. George Parish Community,
Glenolden, Pennsylvania

It is hard to believe, but it will be one year in July since I began the parish nurse ministry at St. George. From the moment I arrived, I felt very welcomed and supported in this ministry. And because of the support I received from everyone in the parish, I have been able to develop programs and workshops tailored to the people of St. George. It is important that the health needs of the parish community are met in a variety of ways, and that is the purpose of my ministry here.

So now I want to take a moment to look back over the year, reflect on the work that has been done, and to consider ways to direct this ministry toward the needs of the people of St. George Parish Community. Like any ministry, the parish nurse ministry needs input and feedback.

When I arrived at the rectory last July 10, I entered an office with an empty desk and an empty computer, but a staff that was eager to see me succeed. And so I hit the ground running! Since that July morning, I have met with many of the parishioners, observed the community, and asked lots of questions. As I learned about the health needs, I have developed several programs to address some of them.

It has been very rewarding to start a blood pressure checking program. Blood pressure equipment was purchased and volunteer nurses provided copies of their licenses, so that we could provide professional services. I want to thank the nurses who volunteered to check blood pressures after Mass on various Sundays throughout the year. In the short time since that program began, we have identified several people who were referred to their physicians and started on blood pressure medicine. We have also affirmed those whose blood pressure is within a healthy range.

I was able to identify several parishioners who needed rides to and from health care providers. Several parishioners volunteered to be drivers for those who needed help.

There are many people within our community who need medical equipment such as wheelchairs, hospital tables, or shower chairs, and there are many people in our community who have such equipment that is no longer being used. We now have a medical equipment donation program in which we can provide medical equipment to those who need it, provided we have it in stock.

During Lent, we held a bereavement lecture in which Rev. Joseph Leggieri, a bereavement speaker, provided encouragement and solace to many of our parishioners who have lost loved ones. Rev. Leggieri spoke from the heart and his own experience to help others find healing and wholeness.

In January, we offered a workshop on long-term care planning. Many of our parishioners are worried about what the future holds and how they are going to be cared for in the event of illness. John DiDonato, Esq., who is a parishioner of St. George Parish, and David McDonald, a social worker, presented valuable and practical information that helped those who attended get a better understanding of the complicated health care system.

I was able to secure the help of the American Red Cross for a certified safe babysitting course. This program was able to help our parishioners provide their own ministry of helping others. We had fifteen girls learn how to provide alert and responsible babysitting, as well as how to appropriately react in an emergency situation. Each girl received a certificate at the end of the class.

As for general health and safety, Mercy Healthcare donated an Automated External Defibrillator (AED). The unit, along with a second one purchased by St. George, will be kept in the church and the parish hall. These units have been proven to improve the survival rate of people who suffer heart attacks when used quickly and correctly. We were also instructed on their use when we presented the parish with a CPR class.

Another very important part of my work here has been to be an advocate for the parishioners. I had the privilege of visiting with many of them and discussing health issues with them. There have been a few occasions when I have had the opportunity to guide parishioners through very confusing health care obstacles. Often our health care problems can be resolved with a few carefully placed phone calls or referrals. It is always a satisfying part of my work to see health care problems resolved or health questions answered.

My first year as parish nurse was filled with many new experiences and exciting challenges. I have seen God's hand guiding us along the way. I am sure there will be many new and exciting adventures for us in the next year. I know that we will grow together in God's love.

Final Word

Clergy who support and facilitate health ministry can have a great impact. Rev. Theodor Fliedner, pastor in Kaiserswerth, Germany, had a great impact on the development of deaconess nursing as a ministry of the church. Fliedner considered the nurse working as a parish deaconess to be as close to the practice of the apostolic church as it was possible to get. His support of health ministry made a huge impact on Florence Nightingale.

Without Granger Westberg's support in Chicago, it is unlikely that wholistic health centers or parish nursing would ever have started in the churches there.

Parish nurses and other lay health ministers need such supporters today, and, indeed, this support among clergy continues to grow. As understanding of the unique aspects of health ministry grows, clergy, health professionals, and other church members are able to see the possibilities this form of partnership can take.

God bless you all.

Appendix A

Budgeting for
Parish Nurse Ministry

First of all, it is important to remember that you are budgeting for a ministry of the church, not funding a parish nurse. This is the church's ministry, not the ministry of an individual, so the church will need to decide how much it wants to invest in this particular ministry. The first step in determining the amount of funding needed for a parish nurse ministry is to assemble a group of people who are interested in participating in a health ministry of the congregation. Often, such a group is called a "health cabinet" or a "health committee."[1]

Once you have this group assembled, ask them to explore the following:

1. What is the role of the church in healing?

2. What are the needs of the community? Consider the needs of seniors, babies, children, families, young adults, middle-aged adults, the hospitalized, those in nursing homes, the homebound, and those with special needs.

3. What is the church doing to serve these needs at the moment?

4. Why would a church want to expand health ministry through engaging a parish nurse?

Once the health cabinet has developed a vision, the next step is to engage the church council or other appropriate groups. If the vision is shared by others in the congregation, then it will be an appropriate time to talk about logistics, including potential costs.

Logistics

Logistics include the following:

1. Is there a nurse in the congregation who is interested in this ministry?

2. Is there a parish nurse network in the area? Often you can find parish nurse networks by calling the spiritual care departments of local hospitals. Your health cabinet might want to explore a partnership with a local network. Start-up funding is sometimes available through these networks, as well as educational preparation and orientation for parish nurses.

3. Will you be paying the parish nurse or providing an honorarium? If so, what are the costs?

Costs

1. *Office expenses.* All parish nurses, paid or unpaid, will need a small office with a desk, a phone with a private, secure answering machine, and a file cabinet that can be locked. A computer would be ideal. Cost: $200 to $2000.

2. *Salary.* Assuming you want to pay your parish nurse, budget an hourly rate less than what you pay your pastor. No joke! Starting salaries for new RNs are generally higher than new seminary grads or many experienced pastors. A good rule of thumb is to pay your parish nurse three or four dollars an hour less than what they would earn as a starting hospital staff nurse. Our parish nurses at Deaconess Parish Nurse Ministries start at $14.50 an hour regardless of degrees held or professional experience, but salaries are higher or lower in other parts of the country. If you work through a parish nurse network, they may set the salary, but even then, it is often negotiable and usually any agreement has a short time period for cancellation (thirty days, for example).

3. *Numbers of hours worked.* Obviously, you are going to pay only half as much for a half-time parish nurse than a full-time

parish nurse at the same hourly rate. Some churches begin health ministries paying their parish nurse for five to ten hours a week, and add hours as the budget grows. A church with a strong commitment to parish nurse ministry is usually able to fund the program long-term even with relatively small membership.

4. *Benefits.* Some parish nurse networks allow you to buy into the group benefits plan for your parish nurse, which is generally far less expensive than a denominational health plan.

5. *Mileage.* Whether the parish nurse is paid or unpaid, the church will probably want to supply mileage reimbursement. Depending on your setting (Boston vs. rural South Dakota, for example), this expense will vary. Range: $600–$1800.

6. *Parish nurse basic preparation.* Parish nurses must be licensed RNs, and there is a course (Parish Nurse Basic Preparation) offered to provide the specialty training. More than 130 Educational Partners of the International Parish Nurse Resource Center offer this thirty-two-hour class around the United States, Canada, Korea, the UK, Swaziland, Zimbabwe, South Africa, Madagascar, Ghana, Australia, New Zealand, the Bahamas, Malaysia, and Singapore. Some of these programs offer the class online. More information on these classes can be found on the IPNRC website, *www.parishnurses.org* (click on "Educational Offerings"). Other preparation classes are offered elsewhere, and interested individuals are urged to select those that provide at least thirty-two hours of instruction. Cost: $475–$1300, depending on whether college credit is earned for the class.

7. *Continuing education.* In the years following the Parish Nurse Basic Preparation class, the congregation should consider setting aside funds for continuing education for its parish nurse. The Westberg Parish Nurse Symposium, sponsored by the IPNRC, and the annual meeting of the Health Ministries Association are both good continuing education resources for parish nurses, and both provide Continuing Education Units (CEUs), (which are needed to meet nursing

licensing renewal requirements in many states). Last year, for example, the Westberg Symposium had over fifty speakers from five continents, all of whom addressed issues of interest to parish nurses and health ministers. Cost: $600 for meeting and hotel (travel extra).

8. *Books and publications.* Two excellent periodicals are produced for parish nurses: *Parish Nurse Perspectives* (available from the IPNRC for $30 a year) and the *Health Ministries Journal* (available from the Health Ministries Association for $59 a year). In addition, several new books on parish nurse ministry appear each year. Cost: $30–$200.

9. *Liability insurance.* The risk of litigation against a parish nurse or a congregation with a parish nurse is extremely low. As of this printing, no parish nurse has ever been found negligent in his or her practice anywhere in the United States, or (to the best of our knowledge) anywhere else in the world. The cost of adding a parish nurse to a church's policy (just as you would add any staff member) is extremely small, generally under $100 annually.

Expense	Range
Office	$200–$2000
Salary*	$0–$30,160
Benefits	$0–$7,500
Mileage	$600–$1800
Basic Preparation Class**	$475–$1300
Continuing Education	$600–$1000
Periodicals/Books	$30–200
Liability Insurance	$100
Total	$2005–$44,060

*Note: Even if the church is unable to pay a salary to its parish nurse, providing a small honorarium as a gesture of recognition of this professional service should be considered.

**Note: Some parish nurse classes are underwritten by grants, so the cost may be as low as "free," but these are not available in all areas. Check with your local parish nurse networks.

Bottom Line

Few parish nurses work full time for one church. Many congregations share a parish nurse between two churches, so the cost for each church with a half-time parish nurse would be slightly more than half of the amounts shown above (each church needs liability insurance, for example, and they may each want to provide an office, depending on location). In some cases, three or more churches have shared a parish nurse successfully, but be aware that while this provides economy of scale in program planning, it reduces the amount of "face time" that a parish nurse can spend with parishioners on Sunday morning, because she or he simply cannot be in three churches at one time. A side benefit of this, though, is that this type of shared ministry tends to bring congregations together. In addition, the parish nurse who is fully employed in his or her profession is able to devote full attention to this ministry without distraction from other employment.

There are many creative ways to support parish nursing ministry. If your congregation is interested in this form of health ministry, one of these ways will be right for you.

Notes

1. For a good resource on putting together a health committee, see the book by Jill Westberg McNamara entitled *The Health Cabinet: How to Start a Wellness Committee in Your Church*, which is listed in appendix E.

Appendix B

HIPAA and Documentation

HIPAA (The Health Insurance Portability and Accountability Act, which was passed by Congress in 1996) speaks to the sharing of private health information between patients, their health care providers, and the insurers who reimburse a portion of the cost of the health care that has been provided. Written in relation to health insurance, it deals with personal health information shared between health care providers and insurers.

Do HIPAA Regulations Apply to Congregations?

There is no direct applicability of HIPAA regulations to parish nurses or clergy serving a congregation unless they seek health information from other health providers, such as a doctor's office or a hospital, or if the parish nurse or clergyperson is an employee of one of those entities. Even in that case, the regulations are not onerous, and should not frighten you or discourage you from continuing your health ministries.

As you would assume, normal standards for confidentiality within the nursing profession apply to parish nurses, and all clergy are encouraged to continue their ethical practices related to sharing of private health information as well. The key is simply an understanding that people do not want anyone to share personal information about themselves with others without their permission. That is easily addressed with a few simple steps.

For example, you may wish to place in your church newsletter a statement such as the following:

In order to protect the privacy of all parishioners, no information about the health status of any parishioner will be sought from another health provider or shared with other individuals by any of the staff members of this congregation without that person's explicit permission.

In most cases, you should not share any health information unless you ask for permission. A good rule of thumb is to ask, "May I share this information with the pastor (or the parish nurse, or the person's son or daughter, etc.)?" Be specific. Ask if the person wants to be remembered in prayer during services and if they would like their particular health concern mentioned.

Must You Always Have Consent?

If, in your professional judgment, a clergyperson or parish nurse believes it to be in the best interest of the parishioner to inform another member of the clergy, the parish nurse, a family member, or a neighbor about a parishioner's health status, then you may share this information without first obtaining the person's permission, but be sure to document this decision.

Under HIPAA regulations you can also release personal health information without the consent of the individual for the following purposes:

- Statutory mandates.

- Hotline calls on behalf of victims of abuse, neglect, or domestic violence. In the case of elder abuse, you have the responsibility under HIPAA to inform the person *for whom* (not against whom) you are making the report, unless you believe that telling them would place them at risk. Be sure to document your call.

- Judicial and administrative proceedings. A parish nurse or clergyperson can ask that the court provide a subpoena for the release of the protected health information if you feel it is in the best interest of the parishioner to withhold it.

- Law enforcement purposes.

- Decedents. For two years after death, medical records are overseen by the estate. After that date, release of personal health information does not require authorization.

- Organ and tissue donation after death.

- Serious threats to health and safety.

- Workers Compensation.

Church Health Records

Parish nurses, like all other nurses in professional practice, are required to keep basic documentation on their professional interactions with those to whom they are providing services. Under HIPAA regulations, someone in a parish nurse's care would be able to request a copy of any health information that is kept about them. Most parish nurses would share a copy of this information as a matter of course, and in an appropriate manner.

A parish nurse should probably ask for a dated, signed statement showing that a copy of the record had been requested and shared with the parishioner, and it is advisable to initial each page of the record so that copies cannot easily be altered.

There may be certain situations, however, when it would be best to deny access. For example, if you are maintaining records in anticipation of litigation, you may deny access to those records. Access may also be denied if it is determined by the patient's physician to be likely to endanger the life or safety of the individual or another person. Also, access may be denied if it is requested by a personal representative and the patient's physician determines that such access is reasonably likely to cause substantial harm.

Often the question is raised, Who owns the records that a parish nurse keeps? In most cases, if the parish nurse is an employee of a health system or other parish nurse program, the records are owned by the employer. If the parish nurse is a direct employee of the church or an non-stipendiary parish nurse, the records belong to the church.

Records must be kept in a secure, locked cabinet, and inactive records must be stored for at least ten years, even if the parish nurse program at the church should end. Health records for children must be kept until the children reach age twenty-one, and any records involved in litigation should be kept for twenty-one years. (It is important to note that there has never been a lawsuit for malpractice filed against a parish nurse — anywhere, ever. There is very low risk in parish nursing practice, because this is not "hands-on" nursing practice.)

Privacy in the Office

Under HIPAA regulations, any conversations between a parish nurse and a parishioner that are related to private health information must be held, to the maximum extent possible, in areas that cannot be overheard by others. If the parish nurse office is in a church library, for example, the parish nurse must be able, during her or his office hours, to have sole use of the room, with the ability to close the door when meeting with people.

Using good ethical standards, the same should hold true for private conversations between clergy and parishioners. Of course, as you know, a window in a church office door is a good thing!

Clergy and parish nurses should have phone lines on which parishioners may leave private messages. If you leave a message on an answering machine about a health concern of a parishioner, you can say the name of the person you are calling and leave your name and number, asking that person to call you back.

If a parish nurse or pastor were to send any e-mails or faxes with personal health information (probably rare), that e-mail or fax must state the confidential nature of the contents and have instructions for its retrieval or disposal should the fax or e-mail be misdirected.

Parish nurses may keep health information on a computer at church or home as long as it is protected by a password that allows entry to those files only by the parish nurse. The password also must be changed on a regular basis and never shared with others. It is advisable that all records be kept at the church, but sometimes this is highly impractical or even impossible for parish nurses. In this case, the same precautions for security of health information should be taken.

Any written materials, such as a calendar, or electronic storage devices, such as a Palm Pilot or Blackberry, that has personal health information recorded must be protected. The health provider (in this case, the parish nurse) is responsible for ensuring that any personal health information remains confidential.

Being There for Your Parishioners

Some things haven't changed at all under these regulations. For example, a nurse or clergyperson (or anyone else the patient designates) would continue to have the right to accompany the patient on any visit with a provider if that patient requests their presence. The same would hold true for hospital visitation: if the patient wants you there, you have the right to be there. There have been instances of confusion as health care providers seek to protect themselves from legal exposure by prohibiting the presence of a parish nurse in health care settings, even when the presence of the parish nurse was requested by the parishioner to help him or her understand the health information being discussed.

The best rule of thumb simply is an ethical sensitivity to another person's privacy. Just because something is legal, doesn't make it ethical. Always ask if you can share information you have been told, and in what ways it can be shared (with the parish nurse or clergy, with a prayer group, with the congregation), and you will be in compliance. The law is no more stringent than good ethical practice, which should be in place in every church at every time.

For a more complete explanation of the standards to protect the privacy of personal health information, visit the website of the U.S. Department of Health and Human Services: *www.hhs.gov/ocr/hipaa.*

Appendix C

Parish Nursing
and Pandemic Preparedness

Jeannie Hill, RN, Project Director,
Health Ministries Network of Minnesota,
and Lori Anderson, RN, Manager of
the HealthEast Parish Nurse Network (HEPNN),
St. Paul, Minnesota

We must build dikes of courage to hold back the flood
of fear.   — Martin Luther King Jr.

The Health Ministries Network of Minnesota has been proactive
about pandemic preparedness. It hosted an event offered by
the Central Minnesota Bioterrorism Hospital Preparedness Program and offered Minnesota's first Faith Community Pandemic
Preparedness Planning Seminar on August 29, 2006, in Sartell,
Minnesota. In a collaborative effort with public health and emergency management, the event was well attended by parish nurses,
church leaders, chaplains, staff of faith-based organizations, and
other community leaders.

Many scientists say it is undoubtedly, "when" not "if," a pandemic will happen, so preparedness is essential. It is clear that all
current response systems would be outstripped; we have before
us an urgent need to build collaborative networks of response.
The faith community has often been first on the scene when
disaster strikes.

Today the role of parish nurses spans the full spectrum of the faith community. Having sprung from Christian roots, the role of parish nurses is being adopted in mosques, synagogues, and many other community organizations. Many of our hospitals were born out of the faithful work of founders from churches or other religious structures. Over time, the connections diminished, and most health care systems now forge connections to faith communities through their spiritual care departments. Alongside hospital chaplains, parish nurses carry forward this vital connection between the medical sector and faith communities.

In 1997, the American Nurses Association (ANA) recognized parish nursing as a needed nursing specialty with clear roles and standards of practice. Primarily, parish nurses help individuals and families take responsibility for their own health and wellness. At the heart of pandemic preparedness is the individual and family need to engage personal responsibility to sustain basic health and wellness if our society is altered by a crisis.

Parish nurses offer hospital staff a source of community support to counter worry with purposeful action. Understanding how faith is central to a positive attitude, parish nurses help others remain hopeful. People in crisis may be immobilized by fear, and such responses must be countered with hope and courage. Hope creates energy and sustains focus, providing a lifeline to one caught in a crisis. Faith community leaders functioning as "dikes of courage" will help keep our emergency rooms free of "worried patients" and available for those truly desperate for medical care.

Parish nurses can assist individuals and families in their faith community in sorting through the pandemic preparedness information. As members of the pastoral staff, parish nurses are positioned to make appropriate referrals to public health and other reliable informational resources. Parish nurses can also assist local congregations in convening preparedness planning workshops. Working to improve one's ability to be self-sustaining in an altered state of society reduces the fear of pandemic. Preplanning reduces vulnerability and sets broader relationships in place for when they are needed.

A pandemic would affect all members of society. Currently, parish nurses are often the source of community care to discharged patients, isolated seniors, the homebound, the handicapped, the chronically ill, and other special needs populations. Parish nurses can work collaboratively to reach individuals on the margins.

Parish nurses, because of their trusted presence, can readily function as point persons in a pandemic situation. Their faith and hope, as living tokens, will go a long way in building the "dikes of courage" needed to face pandemics.

Appendix D

The Church and Organ Donation

Mary Jane Fulcher, RN, MSN, Director,
Congregational Nurse Project of Northwest Ohio

The need for organ donors has never been greater, as the shortage continues to grow at a staggering rate of one American added to the national waiting list every thirteen minutes. More than 97,157 people in the United States are waiting for a life-saving organ transplant and hundreds of thousands need life-enhancing cornea and tissue transplants.[1] The good news is that one donor can save up to eight lives and enhance the lives of more than fifty others.

All major religions support organ and tissue donation. While religious viewpoints may vary slightly, the commonality is that organ and tissue donation is a person's last and final act of charity. Donation is recognized around the globe as an act of profound kindness and can transform a tragic situation into one of hope and new life for a person in need.

A parish nurse can play a vital role in increasing awareness about the need for organ and tissue donors. By reaching out to the congregation through educational programs, community health fairs, and personal visits, parish nurses can encourage others to learn facts about donation and to discuss their wishes with loved ones.

Family members should be aware of each other's desire to donate organs and tissues. Upon death, medical officials, as part of the donation process, will consult the next of kin. While an end of life decision is never easy, by having a family discussion, loved ones will be relieved of making a difficult decision during a very sorrowful time. Addressing the issue of donation could be the catalyst for discussions and lighten the burden of a family. As a trusted member of the congregation, the parish nurse will be asked to address concerns about donation. Common questions include:

• *Will my medical treatment suffer if I decide to be a donor?* No. You are considered a candidate for donation only if you have been declared brain dead. Every effort is made to save the life of a patient.

• *Does donation restrict regular funeral services, including an open casket?* No. Removal of donated organs and tissues occurs during a surgical procedure and the donor's body is treated with dignity and respect, allowing for an open casket funeral.

• *Will my family pay or receive fees if I am a donor?* No. Donor families do not pay or receive payment for organ and tissue donation. It is illegal in the United States (and most other countries) to buy or sell human organs or tissue.

• *Are there age limits for donation?* There are no firm age limits to be a donor. Medical staff will evaluate each potential donor for suitability. There have been donors in their seventies and eighties.

Notes

1. Data from the United Network for Organ Sharing (*www.unos.org*), accessed September 6, 2007.

Appendix E

Books, DVDs, and Online Resources

Books

Chase-Ziolek, Mary. *Health, Healing and Wholeness: Engaging Congregations in Ministries of Health*. Cleveland: Pilgrim Press, 2005.

Clarke, Margaret, and Joann Olson. *Nursing within a Faith Community: Promoting Health in Times of Transition*. Thousand Oaks, CA: Sage, 2000.

Evans, Abigail Rian. *The Healing Church: Practical Programs for Health Ministries*. Cleveland: United Church Press, 2000.

Gunderson, Gary. *Deeply Woven Roots: Improving the Quality of Life in Your Community*. Minneapolis: Augsburg Fortress, 1997.

Hale, W. Daniel, and Harold George Koenig. *Healing Bodies and Souls: A Practical Guide for Congregations*. Minneapolis: Augsburg Fortress, 2003.

McNamara, Jill Westberg. *Health and Wellness: What Your Faith Community Can Do*. Cleveland: Pilgrim Press, 2006.

———. *The Health Cabinet: How to Start a Wellness Committee in Your Church*, 1997. Reprint. St. Louis: International Parish Nurse Resource Center, 2002.

Patterson, Deborah L. *The Essential Parish Nurse: ABCs for Congregational Health Ministry*. Cleveland: Pilgrim Press, 2003.

———. *Healing Words for Healing People: Prayers and Meditations for Parish Nurses and Other Health Professionals*. Cleveland: Pilgrim Press, 2005.

Solari-Twadell, Phyllis Ann, and Mary Ann McDermott. *Parish Nursing: Development, Education, and Administration*. St. Louis: Mosby, 2005.

———. *Parish Nursing: Promoting Whole Person Health within Faith Communities*. Thousand Oaks, CA: Sage, 1999.

Westberg, Granger E., with Jill Westberg McNamara. *The Parish Nurse: Providing a Minister of Health for Your Congregation*. Rev. ed. Minneapolis: Augsburg Fortress, 1990.

Westberg, Granger E., with William M. Peterson, ed. *Granger West-berg Verbatim: A Vision for Faith and Health.* Rev. ed. St. Louis: International Parish Nurse Resource Center, 2002.

DVDs

A Look at Parish Nursing. This ten-minute DVD explores the roles of parish nursing in a congregation, through the eyes of clergy, laity, and parish nurses in several different church settings. With candor and humor, this resource quickly walks a church council, health cabinet, or other group through an introduction to parish nursing as part of a congregation's health ministry. Available through the International Parish Nurse Resource Center at 314-918-2559 or online at *www.parishnurses.org.*

The Spirit of Healing. This film's primary goals are to provide an understanding of parish nursing, to explore the diversity of the nurse's role, and to demonstrate the impact of a parish nurse ministry on healing and health. This DVD has been developed by the Advocate Health Care Parish Nurse Ministry as an educational resource for nurses, clergy, health care systems, and faith communities. To order this DVD, contact Advocate Health Care Parish Nurse Ministry at *denise.dowling@advocatehealth.com* or call 847-384-3744.

Online Resources

International Parish Nurse Resource Center, 475 E. Lockwood Avenue, St. Louis, MO 63119. Telephone: 314-918-2559. *www.parishnurses .org.*

Health Ministries Association, 100 North 20th Street, 4th Floor, Philadelphia, PA, 19103. Telephone 215-564-3484. *www.hmassoc.org.*

Canadian Association for Parish Nursing Ministry, c/o Frances Hudson, RN, Parish Nurse, Coordinator, 56 Thames St., S. Ingersoll, ON N5C 4S9. Telephone: 519-485-3390. *www.capnm.ca.*

Parish Nursing Ministries, UK, 3 Barnwell Close, Dunchurch, Nr Rugby, Warwicks CV22 6QH. *www.parishnursing.co.uk.*

Australian Faith Community Nurses Association. *www.afcna.org.au.*

Australian Parish Nurse Resource Center. *www.apnrc.org.*

New Zealand Faith Community Nursing Association. *www.faithnursing.co .nz.*

About the Author

Deborah L. Patterson is an ordained United Church of Christ minister and executive director of the International Parish Nurse Resource Center and Deaconess Parish Nurse Ministries in St. Louis. She received the MDiv and DMin degrees from Eden Theological Seminary in St. Louis and holds a master's in Health Administration from Washington University School of Medicine. Her health ministry has taken a variety of forms: from serving as pastor in congregations in Missouri and Illinois, to working in health administration at Deaconess Incarnate Word Health System, to health care philanthropy at Deaconess Foundation, to her current work with the IPNRC and DPNM. She has served on the boards of a wide variety of health ministries.

Patterson is the author of *The Essential Parish Nurse: ABCs for Congregational Health Ministry* (The Pilgrim Press, 2003) and *Healing Words for Healing People: Prayers and Meditations for Parish Nurses and Other Health Professionals* (The Pilgrim Press, 2005). She and her husband, Stephen Patterson, a professor of New Testament at Eden Theological Seminary, have two children, Sophia and John.